The Road to Better Health

Feel Better   Lose Weight   Think Clearer

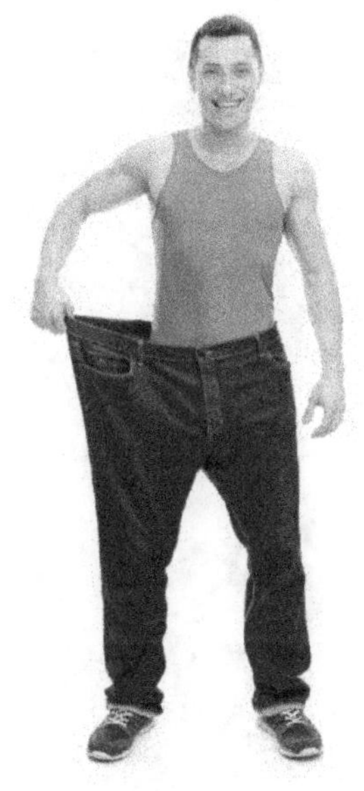

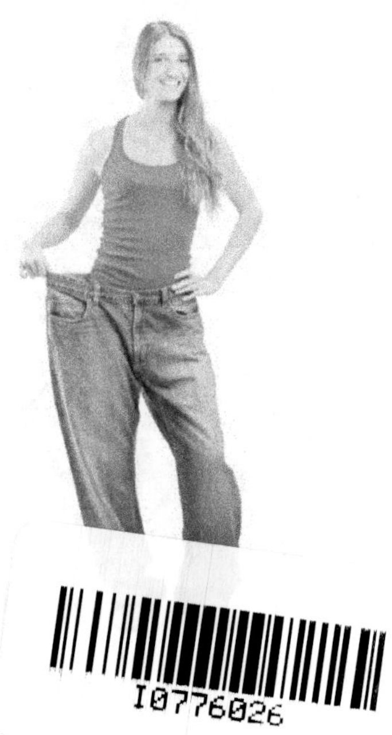

Cary Cavitt

Author & Speaker

To book a speaking engagement please visit us at
www.roadtobetterhealth.net

ISBN-13: 978-1979432573

ISBN-10: 1979432570

Looking for a fun and educational health seminar for your next event?

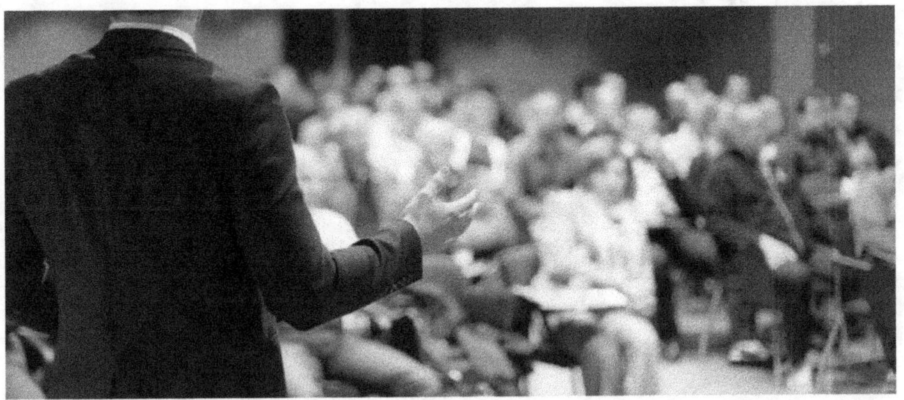

If you would like to book Cary at your next meeting on the topic of improving your overall health, then please visit us at:

www.roadtobetterhealth.net

Whether your next event revolves around offering a health seminar for your workplace, upcoming expo or conference, church or civic club, or any other type of social group, our ***Road to Better Health Seminars*** are a perfect fit to educate your audience *on how to feel better, lose weight, and think clearer.* Contact us today at www.roadtobetterhealth.net.

This book is dedicated to our adult children.

Thank you Sara, Nathan, Phill and Hanna for allowing Mom and I to continue to watch you grow your wings and follow the plan that God has set for your lives. Our prayer is that you will trust Him always.

"If what you are eating is not REAL FOOD, but instead made in a manufacturing plant, then it will be difficult to maintain a healthy body as well as a healthy weight."

- Cary Cavitt

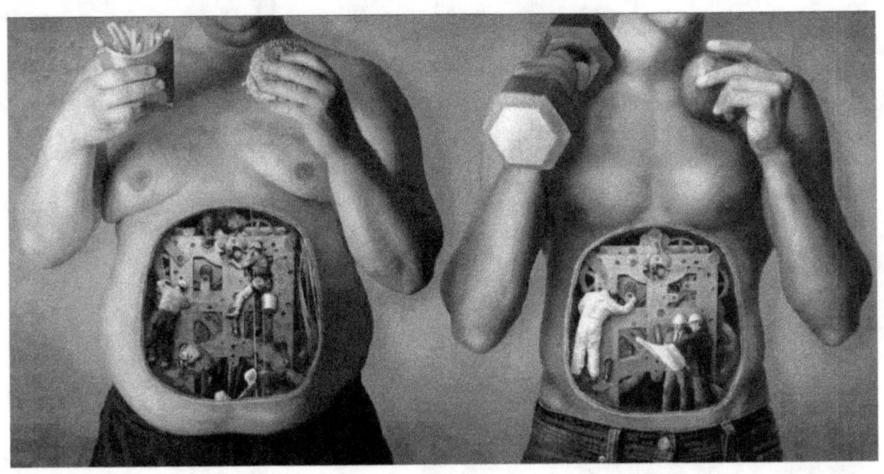

You alone will have the final say on your food choices.

In the final analysis, each person individually will be given the final authority on how he or she will eat. It will also be these personal food choices that will ultimately determine the direction of your overall health.

The foods that we choose to eat will be the #1 deciding factor when it comes to feeling better, losing weight, and thinking clearer.

In my personal opinion there really is only one way to restore a person's health. And that is to eat REAL FOOD.

Table of Contexts

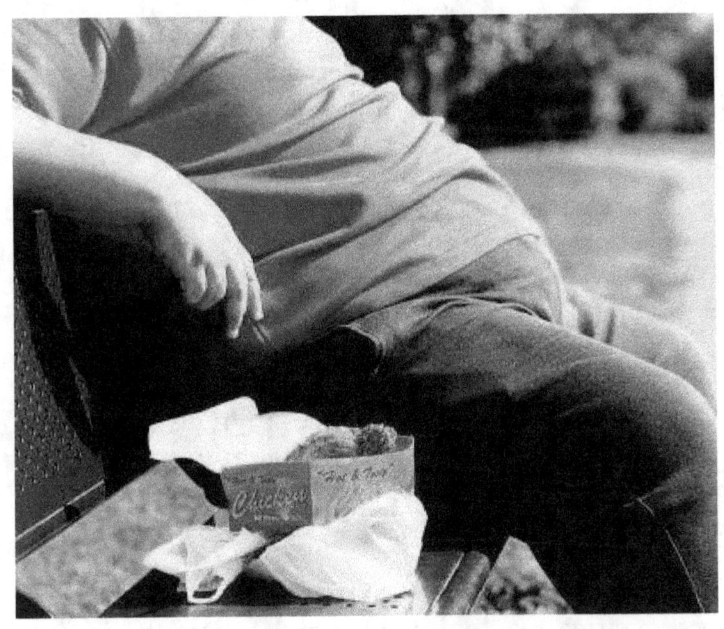

Introduction

Why do I write about how to feel better, lose weight, and think clearer?

Great question and here is my answer. I simply have a heart for those who are either fighting obesity, do not feel healthy, or simply are tired of not being able to lose weight.

What also drives me is witnessing two things that I consistently observe at the gym that continues to feed my passion to share what genuinely will work for the vast majority of people who want to lose weight, regain health, and feel better overall.

The first thing that I have noticed in the gym is the large number of dedicated people who are there with the primary goal of losing weight. Men and women are huffing and puffing on the treadmill or another machine with the single goal of making their hips and bellies disappear.

But losing weight has very little to do with huffing and puffing. Sure the exercise has many great benefits, but losing weight is not one of them. And sure you may lose a few pounds, but that is about it. Please understand that weight loss happens in the kitchen.

The second thing that I notice in the gym is the continual stream of diet program commercials that constantly are playing on one of the dozen TV's hanging from the ceiling promising that you can look like the skinny model that is pushing the latest and greatest diet program for a fee.

In my personal opinion these TV diet programs are nothing more than scams as approximately 98% of them eventually fail in the long run for the average person (only people who love to starve themselves succeed).

What keeps this annual multi-billion business afloat is that they are banking on getting new gullible people to "join the program" and get sucked into a monthly automatic credit card payment. In my opinion it is the new people who join that keeps the boat floating.

And trust me when I say that the TV diet programs are here to stay and will not be going away for a very long time. Most follow the same script in restricting your calories and in the process making you feel miserable after 3-4 months of following their calorie-restricted wonder diet.

So hopefully this answers the question of why I am passionate about sharing what I have learned in fighting the obesity dilemma that is plaguing our society.

My end goal and satisfaction would be to hopefully assist someone out there who may be fighting a health issue or struggling with hidden depression due to a weight problem and desperately wants to lose weight in a safe and healthy manner without having to starve themselves.

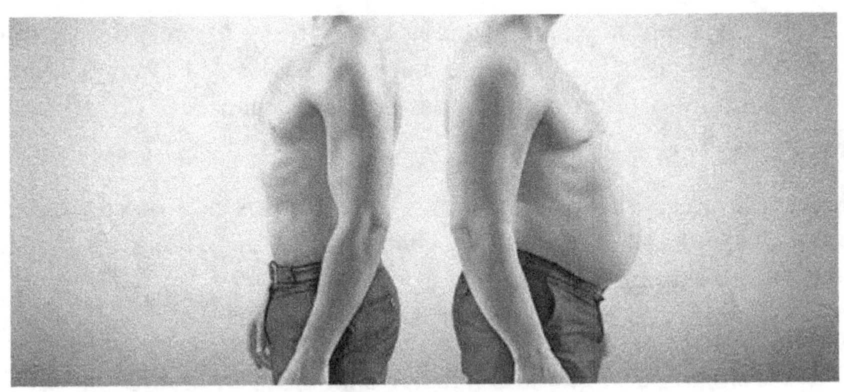

Tip #1
Sugar: The fat elephant in the room

Everyone agrees that we in America have an obesity epidemic that continues to grow year after year with more and more people struggling with weight gain. So what is the reason for this?

Look at any old video clip or picture from the 1940's and 1950's of people living at that time and a high percentage look trim and fit.

Once food manufacturers recognized that this cheap commodity called sugar could make a great food filler (and court our sweet tooth), the overweight epidemic took off at full speed.

It began to occur in the 1960's spearheaded by a man named Ancel Benjamin Keys, an American physiologist who basically vilified fats which gave way to replacing fats with sugar. His false conclusion on fats have since been debunked (simply Google it), but the vast majority of Americas still are in the dark on this subject but continue to accept sugar with open arms.

From there we as Americans went and continue to stay on a low fat diet (thinking we will get skinny), but do not realize that the real culprit to our obesity and disease plague has everything to do with sugar (and not good fats).

The deadly toxin sugar is in up to 80% of any grocery store food item and we as a nation have become ADDICTED to it. Most processed foods (born in a factory) are laced with this fat producing stuff.

Without getting into the reasoning for why this is a poison (again simply Google it), let's just say that sugar is the #1 contributor to getting and staying overweight.

And remember that your body does not know the difference *since sugar is sugar is sugar is sugar.* It shoots up your insulin which then contributes to storing fat in the body (think hips, belly, thighs, etc.).

Just as important is that anything that converts to sugar once it enters your mouth (think breads, pastas, rice, potatoes, snacks, juices, cereals, etc.) also instantly raises your insulin which is a major reason for weight gain and the perfect setting for various diseases.

When our insulin is continually high we spend our day basically burning sugar and carbs (or what I call CARBage). But if we can learn how to keep our insulin LOW throughout the day we are now allowing our body to burn fat off (which then results in weight loss).

Sugar is truly the elephant in the room and so highly addictive. One interesting study was making a group of rats addicted to cocaine. They then put them into a box where there was a pile of cocaine and a pile of sugar. 80% of the cocaine addicted rats ended up rejecting the pile of cocaine and hanging out at the pile of sugar. It is a serious addiction and a toxin we love to have in our system.

The average American consumes around 150 pounds of sugar annually (in 1900 it was 60 pounds). That would equate to approximately 3 pounds of sugar consumed weekly which is terrible for a person's health.

Whether it is in the form of the recognized white or brown sugar, or the 61 hidden sugar names found on an ingredient list in a food label, *sugar is and always will be the culprit to our obesity issue.* Take away this deadly poison and weight will begin to melt.

Creating 61 names for sugar confuses consumers and lowers the odds of recognition. Here are the various names that sugar goes by:

- Agave nectar
- Barbados sugar
- Barley malt
- Barley malt syrup
- Beet sugar
- Brown sugar
- Buttered syrup
- Cane juice
- Cane juice crystals
- Cane sugar
- Caramel
- Carob syrup
- Castor sugar
- Coconut palm sugar
- Coconut sugar
- Confectioner's sugar
- Corn sweetener
- Corn syrup
- Corn syrup solids
- Date sugar
- Dehydrated cane juice
- Demerara sugar
- Dextrin
- Dextrose
- Evaporated cane juice
- Free-flowing brown sugars
- Fructose
- Fruit juice
- Fruit juice concentrate
- Glucose

- Glucose solids
- Golden sugar
- Golden syrup
- Grape sugar
- HFCS (high-fructose corn syrup)
- Honey
- Icing sugar
- Invert sugar
- Malt syrup
- Maltodextrin
- Maltol
- Maltose
- Mannose
- Maple syrup
- Molasses
- Muscovado
- Palm sugar
- Panocha
- Powdered sugar
- Raw sugar
- Refiner's syrup
- Rice syrup
- Saccharose
- Sorghum syrup
- Sucrose
- Sugar (granulated)
- Sweet sorghum
- Syrup
- Treacle
- Turbinado sugar
- Yellow sugar

So what is my advice for those out there who are tired of yo-yo dieting which fails simply because no one likes to starve themselves for an extended amount of time?

My advice is to run as fast as you can from sugar and anything that instantly converts to sugar in your body. Eat REAL FOOD and the elephant in the room will soon disappear.

The first week or two may be difficult simply because of the serious withdrawal that may take place as your body begins to detox from this toxin and desperately scream for a sugar fix.

But if you can begin to learn to eat REAL FOOD (again Google and learn what real food is...what they ate prior to the advent of processed foods), and see sugar for what it truly is, you will begin to not only lose the weight that may have been plaguing you for years, but your health and clarity of mind will drastically begin to improve as well.

If you are serious about improving your health, then set a campaign in your own personal life to recognize this deadly and fattening toxin. *Sugar has zero nutritional value but is simply a cheap food filler* (and profit maker) that is used in most foods.

We only have one body. Learn to avoid sugar and your health and body weight will begin to improve.

"Sugar has zero nutritional value but is simply a cheap food filler."

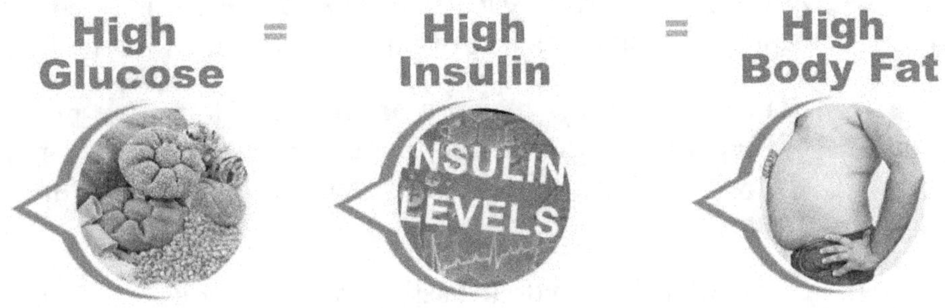

Tip #2
Tired of carrying extra weight

One day earlier this year I stumbled on a YouTube video of a man they call *Butter Bob*. He is just a simple, humble guy from Tennessee who once weighed 320 pounds before dropping to 175 pounds.

This nice guy totally opened my eyes to what has become a total game changer in my own personal health as well as the most important point that I have ever learned in the area of losing weight... and that is gaining a clearer understanding on the damaging effects of having high insulin in your body.

Butter Bob understands why the majority of people are overweight and here are a few points that he clearly articulates in his 15+ YouTube videos:

1. Always having high insulin is the major culprit to storing fat on the body. High Insulin not only stores fat on the body, but also keeps you burning sugar and carbs all day (which is not good for trying to lose weight). Learn to keep your insulin low (with low glycemic foods) and your body will begin to burn fat (which results in weight loss).

2. Stop eating processed foods that always make you hungry soon after (think breads, pasta, rice, potatoes - all spikes the

insulin) and learn to eat REAL FOODS that bring about a happy belly and a feeling of fullness for a very long time.

3. Remember that the majority of processed foods are meant to keep you unsatisfied and that is the reason that you may always feel hungry soon after eating a high carbohydrate meal.

4. Learn what Intermittent Fasting is (just Google it). It is a total game changer and allows our body time to rest instead of constantly filling our belly. By eating daily at a window of time (say 12 pm to 8 pm) we now give our body 16 hours to rest, burn fat, and the means to let go of unwanted fat around the waistline.

All it takes is 26 minutes to watch Butter Bob explain what he (and now I) believes what is one of the major causes of not only obesity, but a whole list of other diseases, and that is having constant high insulin.

Simply go to YouTube and watch Butter Bob's *The Root of Modern Illness - High Insulin.*

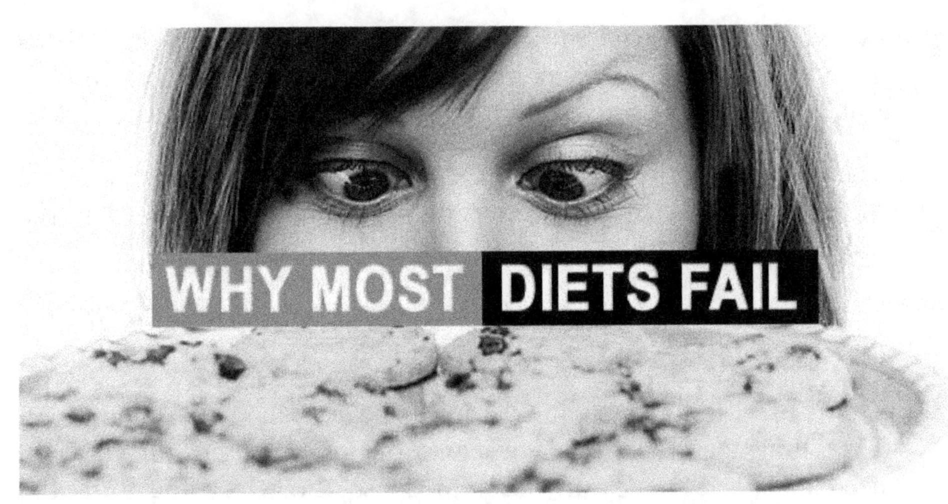

Tip #3
Why most diets eventually fail

The diet industry is an annual billion dollar operation that eventually fails for the majority of those lured in by the TV commercials promising that you can look just like Marie Osmond or any of the other skinny models trying to sell you the latest solution to losing weight.

Commercial after commercial pumps out promises that you can lose weight, but it is going to cost you some cash in the process. It is a big money business and is here to stay as we in America continue to become larger by the minute.

This billion dollar diet industry goes by many names, but basically has the same philosophy behind it: *Restrict your daily calorie intake and weigh will drop.*

And it comes in many names. You can call it Weight Watchers, Jenny Craig, Nutrisystem, or a myriad of other household names that we have all become familiar with through media.

So what is the problem with these calorie restricting diets that show commercial after commercial of heavy people becoming lean?

The real problem with any of these calorie restricting diets is that the vast majority of people eventually fail and lose money in the process.

Here is the typical song and dance example that happens all the time...

Let us use Mrs. Doe as an example. She sees the skinny model on TV telling the world that you can look just like her, but you will need to spend money in order to do so. So Mrs. Doe joins the program and starts her calorie restricting diet, and after 4 months has successfully lost 35 pounds. She believes that she has finally found the golden key to losing weight, and that is to daily restrict her calorie intake.

All of her friends are complimenting Mrs. Doe on her great success, but then month five rolls around and her motivation begins to slowly fade. Mrs. Doe is becoming tired of the program's low daily calorie restriction that is required along with the monthly cash she is forking out.

With motivation gone and finally fed up with always feeling hungry, Mrs. Doe eventually does what millions of other men and women have done prior to her. She quits the calorie restricting program *and the weight eventually comes back with a vengeance.*

She goes back to the popular Standard American Diet (or SAD Diet) and eventually the 35 pounds lost becomes 50 pounds gained.

And here is the real issue in all of this: *The vast majority of us cannot maintain (or stand) a calorie restricting diet.* This is only reserved for the tiny elite who can do this with the gift of having the discipline of a marine. We as humans *do not like* always feel hungry, especially when food is available.

So what is the answer to losing weight without having to follow the typical calorie restricting diet that all of these programs push?

The answer is to stop counting calories and *learn to avoid foods that raise your insulin level.* Eat REAL FOODS that keep your insulin level low throughout the day and you will eventually lose weight and begin to feel much healthier.

Most people live their lives continually in a high insulin state simply because of the foods that they daily consume. *It is high insulin and poor food selections that is the culprit to poor health and weight gain.*

Eat foods that make you feel full and avoid foods that make you feel hungry after 1-2 hours of eating them (think breads, pastas, rice, corn, sugary stuff, potatoes, cereals, etc.). These types of foods instantly raise your insulin level which is not only bad for your overall health, but eventually stores fat on your body.

These television diets really never get to the real culprit of why people are overweight. They all push the same philosophy in that the only way to lose weight is to restrict calories.

Even though this may work at the beginning for those who are motivated enough, eventually the majority will fail because they get sick and tired of basically starving themselves.

If you want to feel full, lose weight, and not have to restrict calories, *learn to avoid foods that instantly raise your insulin.* Google what foods keep your insulin low and you will soon find weight disappearing from your body.

*"The answer is to stop counting
calories and learn to avoid foods that
raise your insulin level."*

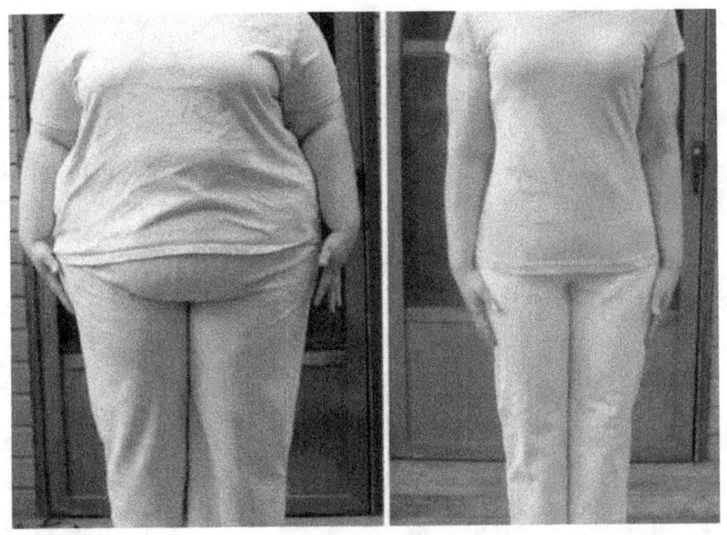

Tip #4
How to become healthy and lose weight

One of the biggest misconceptions that we have been sold for the past 50 years is that fats (meaning good fats) make us fat. Nothing could be further from the truth.

The low-fat, high-carb diet that has been recommended by the mainstream nutrition organizations is a miserable failure and has been repeatedly proven to be ineffective.

Simply Google it as well as look at our current health crisis as we have blindly followed the government's food pyramid chart recommendation which has contributed to our nation's obesity epidemic.

Our bodies need good fats and thinking that these fats are the culprit to poor health or weight gain has been clearly debunked.

The REAL enemy to good health and weight gain is sugar and the addictive processed foods lining our grocery shelves that sadly have become the Standard American Diet (or SAD Diet) for the vast majority in our nation.

We are obsessed and addicted to all of these cheap refined carbohydrate foods (think boxed, bagged, canned or frozen), and this addiction is reflected in our increasingly overweight society.

Since these cheap boxed and bagged foods are readily available (just go to any drive thru), and big profit makers for the giant food companies (think Kraft, Cola-Cola, Pepsi, General Mills, etc.), they are definitely here to stay and will continue to pump out cheap and very profitable manufactured food for the masses.

Bottom line: The Standard American Diet (or SAD Diet) is mainly a diet made up of cheap refined carbohydrates (think breads, rice, corn, flour, pasta, sugary drinks, bagels, cereals, etc.) that instantly converts to sugar in the body, *which is a really bad thing for your health and belly.*

From there your insulin skyrockets and then it needs to store all of this converted sugar, so the insulin does its job and finds a place on your body to place it (think hips, belly, thighs, etc.).

Poor health and weight gain eventually follows simply because our bodies were never meant to live off of these cheap carbohydrate products.

You Can't Out Train A Bad Diet...

Tip #5
Keeping insulin low is the key to losing weight

I was recently speaking with a friend who told me about a man he knows who is trying to lose weight and has decided to hire a trainer to assist him. My friend then asked him about his diet and the man mentioned that he likes his desserts.

Not to burst his bubble, but hiring a trainer to assist in losing his belly is not only a waste of money, but also a waste of time.

Sure exercise is great and commendable, but exercising will do very little to lose the weight that he desperately wants to get rid of.

In reality, the only way to lose weight is in the kitchen and not in the gym. You may lose a few pounds by sweating up a storm with dumbbells and squats, but up to 90% of your weight loss occurs in the kitchen.

If the trainer were smart he would educate this man on *keeping his insulin low* and then it would be much easier get rid of unwanted weight.

He would clearly explain that the culprit to his big belly is due to refined carbohydrates and sugar that raise the insulin, *and as a result stores unwanted fat.*

Get rid of foods that instantly raise your insulin and then you are free to burn your fat as energy (which is the goal for everyone who is trying to lose weight).

Exercise has some great benefits for our overall health, but losing weight should not be our goal in the gym. Only the kitchen ultimately determines this.

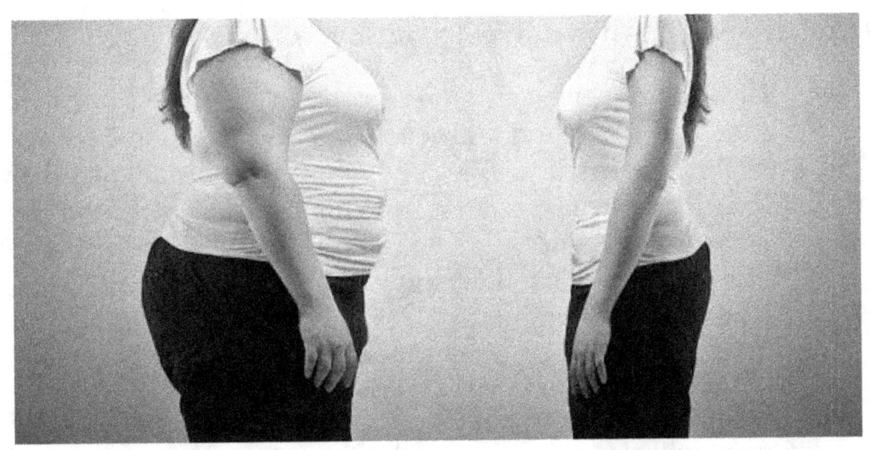

Tip #6
Seven great weight loss tips

Have you ever noticed that almost every diet program being pushed today involves you having to fork over money in order to join? Since it is a billion dollar annual business venture every one of these programs loves to take your money in order to join their *starvation-mode diet* while eating food that is basically terrible for you (think low-calorie pasta, breads, and desserts).

Please do not waste your money on these slick diet TV campaigns since the majority of people eventually fail on them. Sure you may lose a few pounds trying any variety of these TV diet programs, but ultimately most everyone quits simply because people get sick and tired *of restricting their daily calorie intake* and making life miserable.

So what is the answer to losing weight in a more pleasant manner? Simply run from sugar and anything that converts to sugar in your body. These are labeled as food on the shelves and make up around 80% of products in your friendly grocery store. If it is in a box, bag, can or frozen, then the majority of these processed foods are eventually going to put on the pounds.

Here are seven tips if you want to *permanently* lose weight:

1. Run from anything in a box, bag, can, or frozen. Most of these so-called food products are made up of refined carbohydrates that will instantly raise your insulin and then store fat on your body (sorry chip lovers). You may love lasagna but so does your hips and belly. The question you need to ask yourself is this: *would I rather have three minutes of sugar pleasure eating this piece of chocolate cake or have a permanently leaner and healthier body?*

2. Avoid Breads and grains. Eating a slice of whole wheat bread will shoot up your insulin faster than eating a handful of white sugar. Trust me when I say that having a Panera sandwich is terrible for your hips and belly.

3. The majority of boxed foods (did I already say that?). If Laura Ingalls from the *Little House on the Prairie* television series cannot recognize it as being food, trust me, it isn't.

4. So-called health bars. They are nothing more than glorified candy bars. Don't let the packaging with the mountain guy on the wrapping fool you. The majority of these "health" bars will make you fat.

5. Avoid 99.9% of canned or bottled drinks. I am always amazed seeing so many people buying 2-3 cases of soda in the grocery store. Plain and simple it is the large amount of sugar in these drinks that make people become addicted to these poisonous drinks. *And by the way, diet drinks are even worst and are like putting poison into your body.*

6. Avoid all juices, even 100% juices (orange juice, grape juice, etc.). They not only have taken out all of the fiber in the juice, but more importantly will skyrocket your insulin just like that sugar laced Mountain Dew that your cousins in the mountains love to gulp. Move to water if you are a heavy soda or juice drinker, and your waist will soon take notice by slowly disappearing.

7. Eat Good Fats! Your brain is made up of approximately 60% fat. Your body needs good fats *and please do not believe anyone who tells you that fats make you fat.* French fries cooked in vegetable oil makes you fat, but fat from avocados, coconut oil, or meats do not and never have.

Also, my recommendation is to throw away anything in your kitchen with a food label that states *low fat or no fat* since the majority of these factory foods have taken out the good fats and have replaced it with our favorite belly buster toxin affectionately known as sugar.

Dr. Mark Hyman (look him up) wrote a great book entitled *Eat Fat, Get Thin.* If anything else, go to www.amazon.com and read what over 1,000 Amazon readers have said and commented on this topic.

Stop believing what has been clearly debunked, but is still believed by the masses in America. You need good fats in your life *and no, they will not make you fat.*

The real culprit is what the majority of Americans is addicted to but will not confront it head on. Sugar and anything that instantly converts to sugar (think breads, pastas, snacks, corn, rice, cereals, grains, etc.) are the real culprits to our health crisis.

Good fats will not clog your arteries (been debunked). Listed below are some of the manufactured cooking oils that destroy your health and should immediately be thrown out of your kitchen.

Cooking oils to avoid as much as possible:

Canola Oil
Corn Oil
Soybean Oil
Vegetable Oil
Peanut Oil
Sunflower Oil
Safflower Oil
Cottonseed Oil

Stick with Coconut Oil, Olive Oil, and *real butter* as the above cooking oils will eventually damage your health.

Want to change your body from overweight to your ideal weight and feel much better in the process? Educate yourself on the real enemies to weight gain (sugars and refined carbs), and you will *permanently* lose the weight.

Tip #7
Is getting fat a rite of passage as we age?

An interesting question and for most people *they accept it as just a fact of life as we age.* Without batting an eye, the average America over forty just accepts that with age comes more weight to our body.

To set the record straight, gaining weight as we age is really about the *choices of food* that we have made a habit of eating throughout the years. The time of reaping eventually arrives in the form of weight gain.

Here is how it works...

In our teeny bopper years we somehow get away with eating tons of junk food simply because our young and active metabolism allowed us to eat anything we wanted without affecting our hips and waistline.

But as we age all of the sugar and processed foods that we have consumed over the years begin to break down our body and our trim youthful figure slowly begins expanding.

Listen, it is not your metabolism that is the problem. It is that you have not *changed the oil in your car (body)* for the past fifteen years that has damaged your body. All of that sugar is now expanding your body and unless you change your eating habits you will continue to gain weight.

If you are content with being overweight, then all the more power to you. But if you honestly dislike carrying around those extra pounds, want to feel young and healthy again, and have tried everything but nothing seems to work, here are two tips that I recommend:

1. Divorce Sugar
    Sugar is the #1 culprit *to all weight gain.* Our bodies were never meant to consume up to 150 pounds of sugar annually (compared to just 7 ½ pounds consumed on average in the year 1700). It does not matter if it is white or brown sugar, honey, agave sugar, or the dozens of other hidden names of sugar out there since they all react the same to your body. Sugar consumption will assist in storing fat on your body by keeping your insulin high.

2. Divorce Refined Carbohydrates
    The average American consumes a large percentage of their daily calories from refined carbohydrates which is absolutely unhealthy and will eventually make a person overweight.

More importantly, these cheap foods *(but very profitable for the big food companies)* instantly convert to sugar once they are consumed in the body, helping to raise insulin and then store fat on the hips and belly.

You may think you are doing well by avoiding white sugar and obvious unhealthy products, but the real culprit is all of the added sugar *hidden in another name* that you may be consuming and are completely unaware of.

So here is a short list of foods that will not only make you overweight, but also keep you nice and plump in your later years:

a. All Breads / Grains... Trust me when I say that the breads today are a totally different breed and not only will keep you hungry soon after consuming, but eating any kind of bread as a daily source of food will pack on the pounds. Also, why does the average bread label in a store show a long list of ingredients...seriously?

b. Pasta... Sorry Olive Garden lovers. Any and all types of pasta *instantly converts to sugar in your body*, spikes your insulin high, and then is stored as fat on your body.

c. Corn... Corn is in most everything and used as a cheap filler to so many foods out there. And remember, farmers use corn to fatten their cows. Need I say more?

d. All canned drinks... If you drink anything from a can or bottle 99.9% of the time it is terrible for you. Whether it is called a soda, a fruit drink, or a myriad of other names, the vast majority of these canned drinks instantly spikes the insulin and assists in storing fat on the body. The better solution would be to simply drink water.

e. Anything in a box... Stop buying foods from a box as the majority is nothing more that refined carbohydrates that will eventually store fat on your hips and belly. Most boxed foods should be renamed "Fat Storing Stuff." Seriously, *how can anyone call Mac & Cheese a food?*

Simply put, piling on the pounds as we age is really a choice each person individually has to make. And do not let anyone fool you into going on a silly calorie restricting diet that in the end will fail and make your life miserable.

By just *divorcing sugar and all refined carbohydrates* you will soon begin to notice a new you in the mirror that somehow disappeared over the years by innocently following the Standard American Diet (or SAD Diet).

"By just divorcing sugar and all refined carbohydrates you will soon begin to notice a new you in the mirror that somehow disappeared over the years by innocently following the Standard American Diet (or SAD Diet)."

Tip #8
Sugar is killing us and making us fat

When I was in fifth grade my friend Pat and I went to a carnival where we paid a couple of quarters to go behind a curtain and view an overweight lady sitting on a chair just staring back at us. It is sad and amazing that they allowed this to happen at carnivals back in the early 1970's.

What is even sadder is that you do not have to go to a carnival in today's age to see an obese person. Just head to the mall or any local store and you are sure to see quite a few little motorized scooters with large people sitting in them. It is a sad but a true reality within our culture.

My heart goes out to these folks simply because life can be very difficult when someone is fighting obesity. Our quality of life suffers as we cannot enjoy the simply things like walking in the park or a wide assortment of other activities that healthy people take for granted.

If I had the opportunity to talk to anyone who is suffering from obesity my #1 advice would be to remove any and *all types of sugar from their diet* as well as *all refined carbohydrates* that also turn into sugar once it is digested into the body.

I would then help the person to understand that more than likely his or her real problem is a hormonal issue and then tell them that their health would instantly improve if they only understood that having high insulin throughout the day (by bad food choices) could be the real culprit behind their weight gain.

Finally, I would explain to an obese person that their weight will improve if they simply break free *from sugar and refined carbohydrates* and began eating foods that will keep their insulin low throughout the day. This would then allow fat to be burned as the main energy source (what everyone wishes they could do).

There is an answer to obesity and that is to get rid of the addictive toxin known as sugar and processed foods.

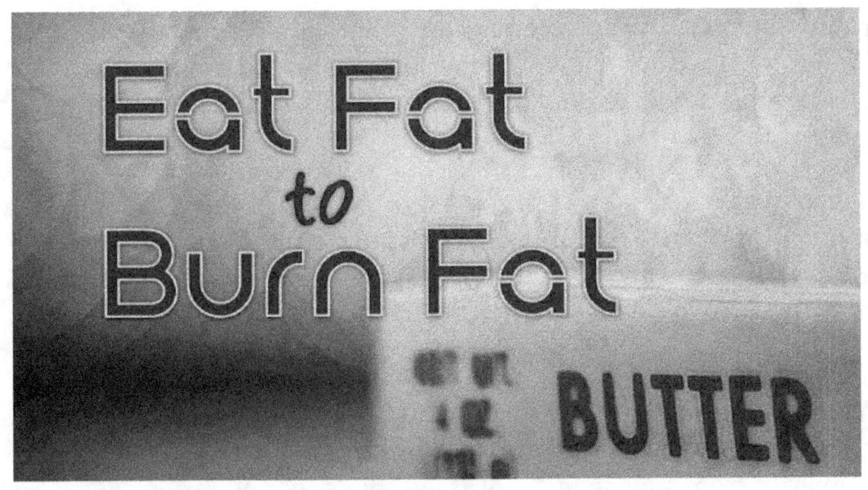

Tip #9
Stop starving yourself if you want to lose weight

The majority of people think that in order to lose unwanted weight they must go on a diet that restricts calories which then makes them live miserably in a starvation mode during the duration of their diet.

It is the complete opposite of what I would recommend if you sincerely want to lose weight *and permanently keep it off.* You will never have to starve yourself and will always feel satisfied.

Here is what I would recommend to anyone wanting to lose weight without the suffering that the majority of these calorie restrictive diets make you go through:

Eat REAL FOOD that has not been manufactured or created in a lab. Real food can be described as food that does not make you hungry again soon after consuming, but genuinely makes you feel completely full after a meal for a very long time. It would be similar to the food that Abe Lincoln may have eaten.

More than likely your ancestors ate real food and did not stuff their bodies with the myriads of refined carbohydrates and sugar laced boxed processed foods found in almost every aisle at you friendly grocery store.

When you eat foods with good fats *(which are great for losing weight),* you will feel full for a very long time. As a matter of fact, you will not want to eat for a long time because good fats completely make you satisfied and in turn greatly assist in losing weight.

You need to reprogram your mind with the fact that good fats will not and have never made anyone fat. The fat on our bodies come primarily from sugars and processed foods, period.

This whole notion that good fats make you fat has been totally debunked. Simply Google this and educate yourself on this topic. If anyone tells you that all fats make you fat please run from them as fast as you can.

On a personal note I use to think eating good fats would make me fat as well until I educated myself. Not only do I attempt to eat the majority of my meals with good fats on my plate, but my overall health has completely improved since I divorced myself from sugars and refined carbohydrates and fell in love with good fats.

This knowledge was a total game changer and I am convinced that any person can lose unwanted weight if they only understood the importance of eating HEALTHY FATS and divorcing themselves from sugar and processed foods.

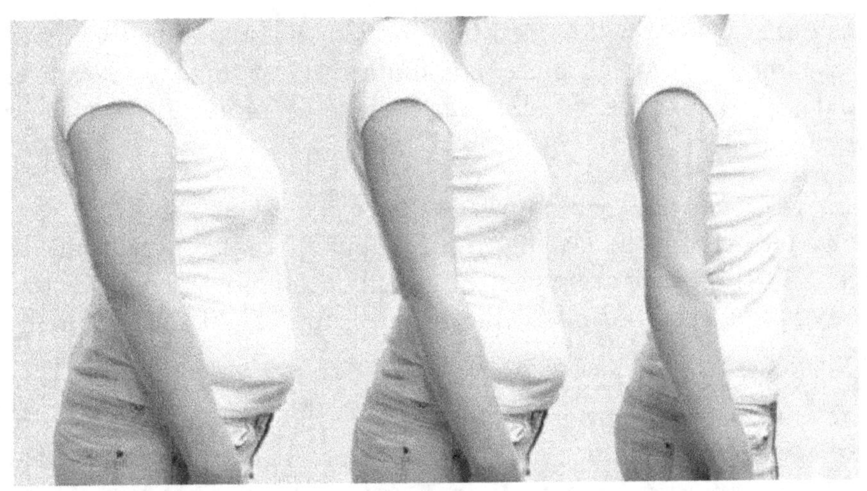

Tip #10
How to get rid of a belly

Go to any gym and you are sure to find both men and women doing sit-ups, crunches, and a host of other core exercises with the desperate hope of shrinking their belly. They grunt and sweat hoping that when they walk out of the gym their belly fat will magically disappear.

Nothing could be further from the truth and this approach to losing belly fat will not and never has worked. Sure you can get a stronger core and these exercises can be great for your back and overall health, but losing the belly fat will never happen.

You see, the only way to lose that belly is performed in the kitchen, period. You can do a billion crunches at the gym until you are blue in the face, but about 90% of belly weight loss can only happen by getting rid of sugar and the hundreds of processed food box products on the market that instantly convert to sugar, and hence makes us fat.

Here is the deal. You or I cannot "spot" fat loss. Weight comes off first in areas such as our face, neck, and arms. Usually the last place that weight will come off is in the belly area. Since we have those important vital organs behind our belly, it somehow wants to hold fat as long as possible as a layer of protection for these organs.

This is where patience comes in. Trust me when I say that your belly fat may be the last fat to leave, but it will eventually take a hike. By simply divorcing sugar and all of the processed foods that convert to sugar and spike your insulin, your weight and eventually your belly will slowly disappear.

Am I opposed to working out and doing those crunches and core exercises? Absolutely not. Exercise is great and has some great benefits, but losing weight is not one of them. That is reserved primarily in the gym called the kitchen.

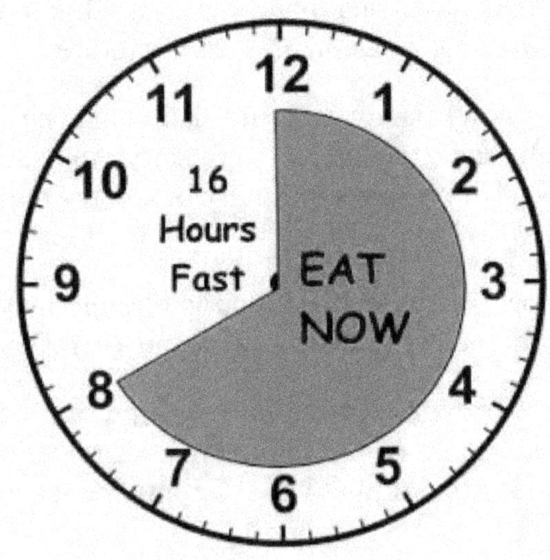

Tip #11
Why I recommend divorcing breakfast

Trust me when I say that you will not die if you stop eating breakfast and that *breakfast is not the most important meal of the day*. Nothing is further from the truth and more than likely Mr. Kellogg, Captain Crunch, and Tony the Tiger has brainwashed our society into believing this fallacy.

I am also quite confident that you have eaten breakfast all of your life and cannot imagine going without it. To even hint that we do not need breakfast has to be classified as heresy to many people.

Listen carefully. At one time breakfast *(which consisted of real food)* may have been important for the majority of people 150 years ago who worked hard and long hours on a farm doing serious all day manual labor. But those days are far gone as we now sit at our desks getting fat with an Egg McMuffin in our hand.

A little history... when our forefathers came over they wanted to be more dignified and separate themselves from other less civilized societies who had no eating plan. So our dignified forefathers invented this *"must eat three meals a day"* culture.

Breakfast was now firmly set in place and now we are all brainwashed into believing that we will starve to death if we do not feed our bellies with pop tarts or a fatty blueberry muffin first thing in the morning.

So what is my beef with breakfast and is it really necessary? In the simplest terms let me give you my two cents on the subject.

When we hit the bed we all eventually go into a *fat burning mode* after about a few hours of sleeping. This is great since being in a fat burning mode is the ultimate goal for anyone wanting to lose fat from their body.

We eventually wake up feeling great and still in that wonderful fat burning mode state. The goal now is to maintain this *fat for energy mode* for as long as possible.

But what do the majority of people do? They quickly break this *wonderful for your health and weight loss fast* by stuffing their face with poor quality food (sorry bagels and breakfast bars) thinking that they will starve and could even possibly die if they have not eaten by noon.

Listen carefully to what I am about to say. If you simply give your body 16+ hours a day to rest from food each day you will not only lose weight, but your overall health will drastically improve.

This is what is referred to as *Intermittent Fasting* which will prolong your fat burning mode and provides many additional health benefits, including fat loss. If you struggle with occasional brain fog, Intermittent Fasting will soon clear it up as well and allow your brain to think more clearly.

Our bodies and digestive systems welcome this time to rest and heal from constantly having to work. I am also convinced that the majority of people in our *'food is everywhere culture'* never experience true hunger simply because they are always stuffing themselves.

In my personal opinion Intermittent Fasting *is one of the absolute best moves anyone can make for their overall health.* Humans were not meant to continually feed themselves with a constant stream of food. But because food is readily available, we do not have the discipline to stop for a short period to allow our body and digestive system to rest.

Trust me as you may dislike the first week or two of not eating breakfast, and your stomach will whine demanding Captain Crunch or one of those breakfast bars that you have consumed for years erroneously thinking they will help you lose weight. But trust me when I say that all of these *made in a factory* bars are detrimental to your health.

I know that you have been taught since kindergarten by your kind teacher to make sure to eat breakfast as this is the most important meal of the day. But this is a manufactured lie brainwashed in our society by the multibillion dollar a year breakfast food companies.

Bottom line: You will not die if you stop eating breakfast. Eat REAL FOODS each day and you will wake up not feeling hungry for a very long time.

On a personal note I am never hungry when I wake up simply because I eat real foods that keep me full for a long period of time *(think good fats).*

Once you get past the first two weeks of listening to your belly moaning and complaining that it did not get its sugar fix *you will never want to go back to eating breakfast again.* Your shrinking belly and overall health will also thank you for it.

"Our bodies and digestive systems welcome this time to rest and heal from constantly having to work. I am also convinced that the majority of people in our 'food is everywhere culture' never experience true hunger simply because they are always stuffing themselves."

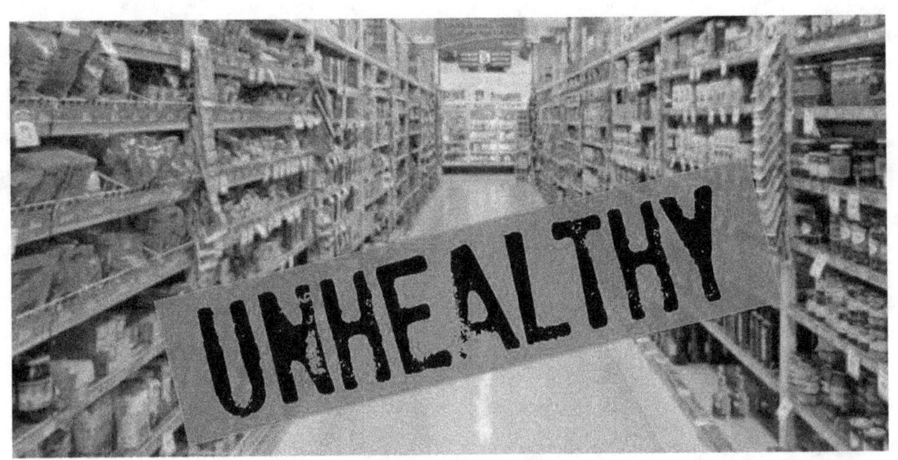

Tip #12
Answer one simple question to lose weight

Here is one simple question that will instantly allow you to make better food choices and lose unwanted weight:

"Would Abe Lincoln have the opportunity to eat this food I am about to put in my mouth?"

If your answer is no then please throw it in the trash can as quickly as possible.

It is a simple but profound question and will instantly make you smarter with what foods that you choose to eat.

Here is a sampling of foods ol' Abe surely did not eat (simply because they had *real food* back then):

Pop tarts
Lasagna
Mountain Dew
Gatorade
Bagels

Chips Aloe
Frosted Flakes
Donuts
Sugary BBQ Sauce
Starbucks sugar loaded drink
Mac & Cheese
French Fries
Boxed anything
Muffins
Soup laced with sugar
Lunchables
Doritos
Greased soaked potato chips
Vegetable & Canola Oil
Cheez-its
Captain Crunch
TV Dinners
and a zillion other boxed or bagged products at a grocery store.

Bottom line: Ol' Abe ate *real food*.

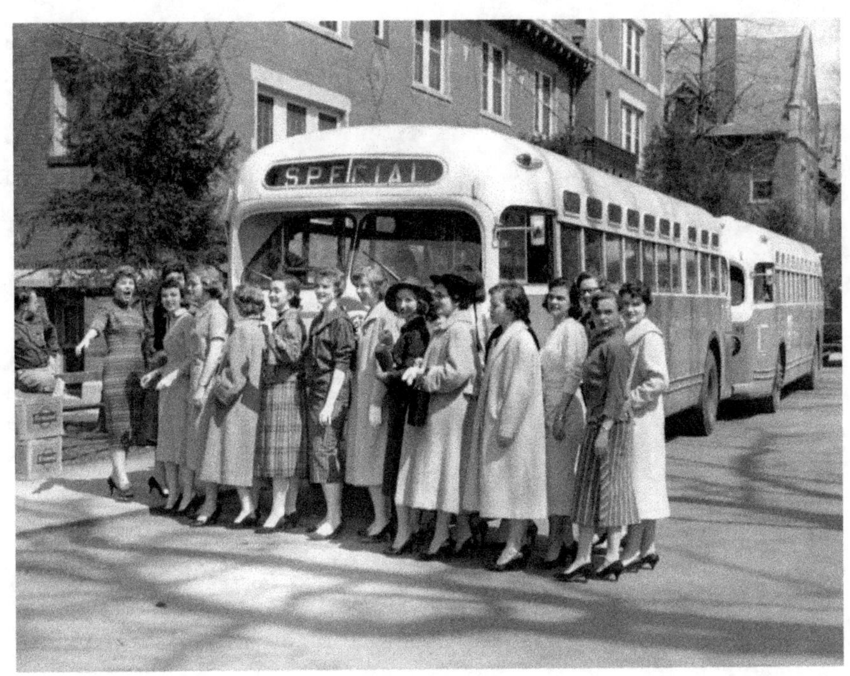

Tip #13
Before the advent of processed foods

Have you ever noticed old pictures from the past prior to the age of *sugar laced everything* and how healthy the majority of people in these vintage pictures looked?

Not only was it rare to see a group picture of overweight people in these older photos, but the majority of pictures reveal a much healthier and leaner society where obesity was a rare occurrence.

Remember that the bottom line with all big food corporations *(think Kraft, General Mills, Coca-Cola, etc.)* is to make big profits, and they do this by making their boxed, bagged, canned, and frozen food taste super yummy by their chemists in white lab coats.

The secret sauce for the majority of their processed manufactured products *is sugar and/or refined carbohydrates* (which converts to sugar in the body).

This fact alone is the #1 reason that we have grown into an overweight nation.

Take away the sugar and their products would sit on the shelves.

Tip #14
Good fats satisfy, but sugar makes you hungry

Why is it that so many people are always hungry soon after eating? It is as if they are never satisfied after eating a meal.

That use to be me. My wife would make us a beautiful lasagna dinner and guess what I would do right after sitting down to this lovely meal? I would get straight up and head to the cereal cabinet in the kitchen and then have one or two bowls of cereal!

Amazing isn't it? But here is the reason why my belly was craving more:

Processed foods never fully satisfy simply because they are not REAL FOOD. These cheap foods end up making us always hungry and eventually put on the pounds.

Sure you may "feel full" after eating a carb rich plate *(think pastas, breads, potatoes, etc.),* but the "feeling full" sensation soon disappears and your belly and brain starts protesting for more food shortly afterwards.

Understand this important point: *Refined carb foods (sorry pasta) only satisfy for a very short time and then tells our brain to eat more of this made in a factory food.* These types of foods go into our system and soon convert into sugar which then makes us crave more of these cheap carbs within an hour or two. What eventually follows is weight gain.

In other words, anything that instantly converts to sugar in our body and raises our insulin *(think refined carbs and boxed foods)* will only make us crave more shortly after consuming because of the sugar effect that it has on our body.

On the other hand, if you replaced these carb rich meals with real food *(think of foods Abe Lincoln may have eaten),* you will not only start to lose weight, but your tummy will feel fully satisfied for a very long time (which is a really good thing).

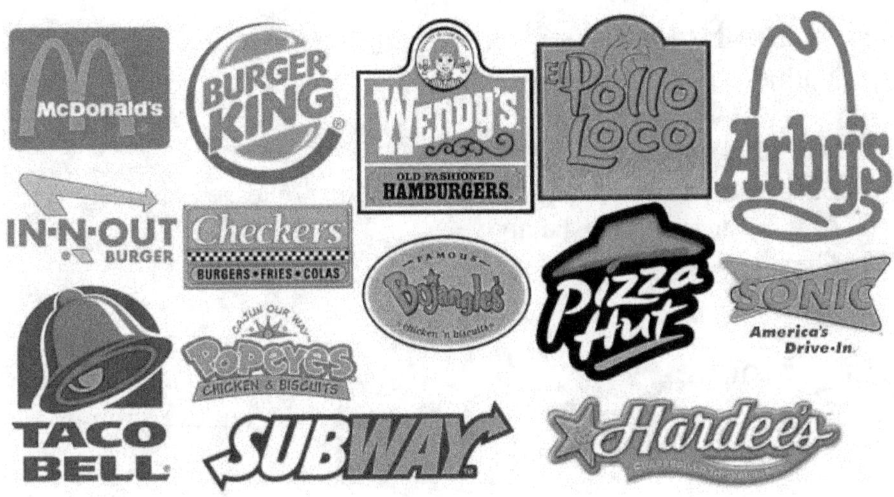

Tip #15
What I would eat at a fast food restaurant

A question that I get asked is *what do you eat?* Here are a few quick thoughts on what I would eat at the various fast (or is it fat?) food restaurants that populate every corner of our great land.

In total honesty, it is my last choice, but sometimes I am stuck and there are no other options to fill my belly.

A. McDonalds

Every once in a while I am at an airport and old Mickey D's is the only choice that is available. So here are a few items that I would choose:

1. The salads that they have (no croutons) with grilled chicken.
2. Eggs & any of the meats
3. Water
* Note: French fries are not even a thought.

B. Taco Bell
1. Nothing (it all goes to the hips and belly)

C. Wendys
1. Baconator without the buns, ketchup, or processed cheese.
2. Any burger without the above
3. Their salads
4. Water

D. Chipotle
1. Bowl with steak or chicken, no rice or beans, but everything else. Lots of good guacamole!

E. Panda Express
1. Steamed Veggies and Chicken (try to avoid the sauces as they are nothing but glorified sugar which eventually contributes to a big belly).
2. Water

F. Every other burger joint:
1. Any burger (the more meat the better), with everything except ketchup, buns, and processed cheese. Avoid the fries & onion rings as they will convert to fat on your body.
2. Always just water.

G. Chilis
1. Steak and broccoli (avoid the potato and just ask for extra broccoli).
2. Some of their salads
3. Burgers without the bun & ketchup
4. Water

H. Subway & Panera
1. Nothing but the salads (bread sandwiches will put on the weight)

I. KFC or Popeyes
1. Nothing but possibly the grilled chicken.

J. Giordano's or the other pizza joints

1. Will eat Giordano's if I am with my family & friends *(but remember ALL pizza breads make us fat & the sauce is mixed with sugar in order to make us keep coming back).*
2. Their salads.

K. Olive Garden

1. Steak or Chicken
2. Salads & Steamed vegetables
* Avoid bread sticks that instantly convert to sugar in the body, raises the insulin, and makes you get brain fog soon after consuming.

L. Starbucks

1. Nothing except tea or black coffee if I were a coffee drinker. All of the dainty food and desserts that Starbucks offers all convert to fat on your body.

I can usually go into any restaurant and find something halfway decent to eat without having to poison my belly with added sugar and refined carbohydrates *(which are most items on a typical restaurant menu).*

And of course there are times when celebrating with family and friends where I may share a no-no food or dessert so I won't be tagged as *"that guy"*.

But trust me when I say this:

The longer you get away from the greasy fries, ice creams, pizzas, breads, sauces, pastas, and all of the other poor food choices that pack on the weight, *your desire for these fat foods will soon disappear* and you will begin to feel better and lose weight simply because you are now eating real food!

"The longer you get away from the greasy fries, ice creams, pizzas, breads, sauces, pastas, and all of the other poor food choices that pack on the weight, your desire for these fat foods will soon disappear and you will begin to feel better and lose weight simply because you are now eating real food!"

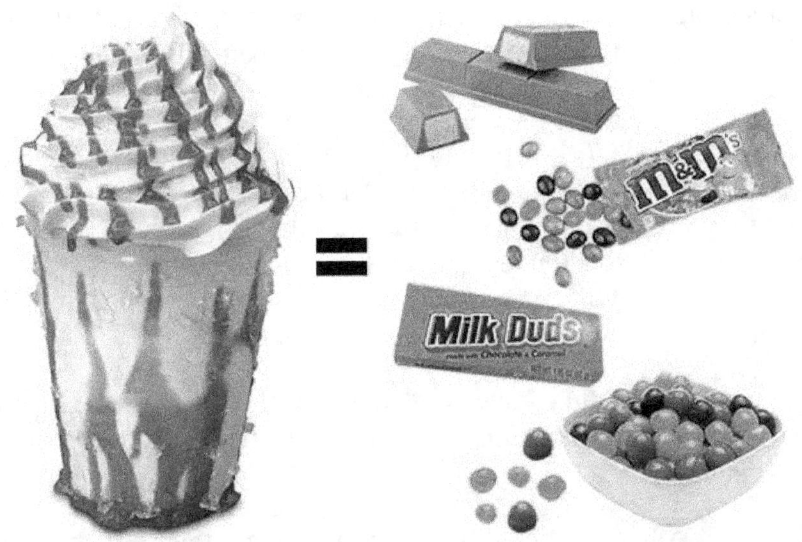

81 GRAMS OF SUGAR IN A CARAMEL FRAPPUCCINO

Tip #16
Starbucks will eventually make you fat

I recognize that I am trending on thin ice to even dare write about the billion dollars a day sugar fix pit stop and comfort zone to a large segment of our adult population.

But it really does not matter what you put sugar into since any and all forms of sugar will eventually make you overweight.

So unless you are one of the disciplined few who get your daily morning Starbucks fix with a plain black coffee or tea, the majority of the drinks offered there are nothing more than glorified desserts.

Also, any of the cute sandwiches or beautiful dainty muffins that they offer will also go straight to your hips.

But seriously, there is a large population out there who has become highly addicted to sugar, and there is no better way to get this fix than from the convenience of a Starbucks drive thru.

Whenever I see a skinny young guy or girl with a Starbucks cup in their hand sipping on a yummy Caramel Frappuccino I imagine that they are not going to like the way they look in a mirror by the time they hit the tender age of thirty. The fun and sugar laced Frappuccinos will eventually settle and put weight on these innocent teeny boppers down the road.

I have absolutely no issue whatsoever with coffee shops operating and making a profit. This is the freedom that has built and made our nation great.

But what concerns me is that the profits are coming *at the expense of loading sugar into the bodies of innocent customers* who have become addicted to sugar and sadly are clueless to this fact.

Of course the same can be said about ice cream shops, candy makers, and the rest of the companies who largely depend on sugar addictive people to buy their sugar laced products.

Imagine for a moment that any and all brands of candy were suddenly banned from using any form of sugar. I can guarantee that every candy company in the world would close their doors within a week. *It is the sugar in the candy that we crave more than anything else.*

So if a Starbucks cup in your hand brings a sense of comfort to you then by all means enjoy it to the max. But just remember those innocent little sips will eventually expand into a not so innocent waistline.

Here is a bonus tip…

Want $202,137.00 in Your Bank Account?

Let us say that you and your wife go to Starbucks five times a week and average spending around $40.00 each week. That would come to about $2,000.00 annually that you are giving to our beloved Starbucks.

Now let us say that you do this annually for 30 years straight. That would be giving Mr. Starbucks a total of $60,000.00 to enjoy their sugary drink as well as provide you with an extra spare tire around the waistline.

But let's turn the table around by imagining that instead of spending the $2,000.00 a year at Starbucks you decide to invest this amount annually for 30 years into say a Vanguard Roth 500 S&P Index fund that wielded an average of 7% annually.

Did you know that after 30 years your $60,000.00 total investment would grow to $202,137.00? Not only would you be able to buy that pretty pink Cadillac that you have always dreamed about, but you would have a much smaller waistline in your later years!

"What concerns me is that the profits are coming at the expense of loading sugar into the bodies of innocent customers who have become addicted to sugar and sadly are clueless to this fact."

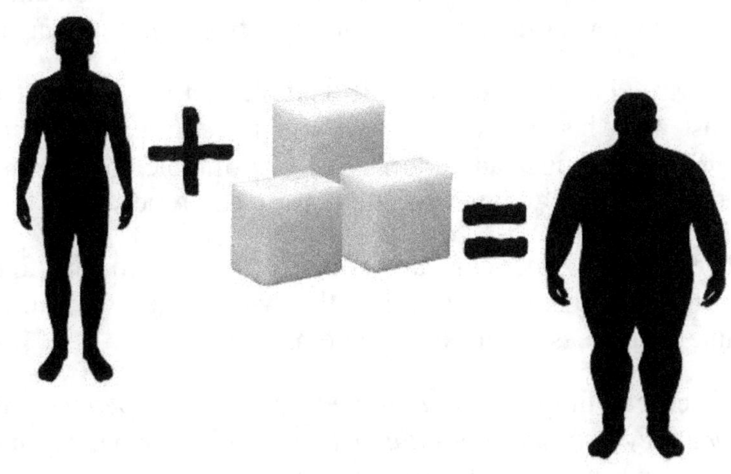

Tip #17
Sugar is the culprit to your overweight problem

No matter how you slice or dice it, the number one reason that you are fighting a weight issue *is due largely to the dangerous toxin innocently known as sugar.*

It is everywhere and in everything, and is the most important guest at every celebration that occurs on the planet.

Go to a park and a cute little ice cream truck is innocently pedaling our little friend hidden in all of those yummy ice cream treats. Guzzle down a soda pop and you are instantly rewarded with nine teaspoons of sugar.

That beautiful cake at your nephew's fifth birthday party is filled with the magical substance that we love to put into our mouth in order to get an instance sugar fix. It soon rushes through our blood stream and gives our brain that sugar high *that we have unknowingly became addicted to.*

So what if soon afterwards we have to loosen our belt and get brain fog for a few hours after enjoying this five minute sugar rush.

It is true but very few want to believe that sugar is that bad. But trust me when I say that *sugar is the real culprit to our obesity epidemic.* Sugar addiction is very profitable for the major food companies and will not be going away any time soon.

The average American eats around 150 pounds of this toxin in one form or another every year and then we wonder why our nation has an ever increasing obesity problem.

Listen carefully. *Sugar is addicting and most people are clueless that they are actually addicted to it.* We rationalize since it is a legal substance and our government has put their stamp of approval on it. So surely it must be safe for us, right?

So what is my take on this pleasurable chemical called sugar? I personally feel that the primary suspect for our nation's health epidemic and obesity issue is caused by sugar *first and foremost.*

I am also convinced that if people divorced themselves from this addictive substance, not only would our nation's health instantly improve, but all of those extra pounds would soon melt away.

But because sugar is everywhere and in everything, the goal to get it completely out of your own personal life will feel like a constant uphill battle. *Very few in our society cannot or will not divorce from sugar simply because they love the brief pleasure that it offers.*

And the temptation is everywhere. You can be at the grocery store checkout innocently picking up some eggs and all of a sudden your favorite candy bar is staring right at you next to the cash register. You then begin recalling all of the fond and joyful memories of getting a sugar high with this innocent candy bar.

It is so tempting to want to buy that peanut butter cup and get five minutes of sugar bliss. Your whole body begins screaming for the instant pleasure that it will bring. Anyways, it is a rainy day and an innocent little sugar pleasure would sure lift the clouds for a brief moment.

But be warned if you want to get out of your relationship with sugar. Once it finds out that you are leaving it will soon find subtle and covert ways to get you back. *Will you have the strength and courage to be different* from the masses that would never dare think of leaving their secret best friend?

The bottom line really comes down to the choice of whether you really want to lose all of that extra weight on your body, or if you would rather continue to stay with the little culprit that made you overweight in the first place.

You alone will have to make that choice.

"The bottom line really comes down to the choice of whether you really want to lose all of that extra weight on your body, or if you would rather continue to stay with the little culprit that made you overweight in the first place."

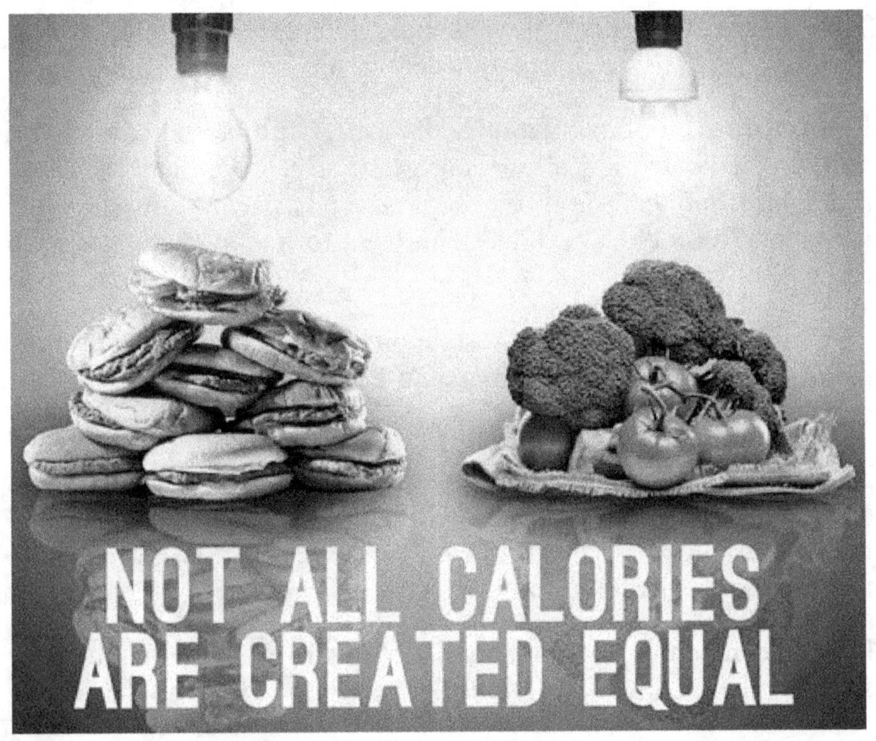

Tip #18
Exposing the calorie myth: A calorie is not a calorie

There is a completely false premise floating out there that *a calorie is a calorie.* Nothing could be further from the truth.

Of course big food companies would love for you to believe this lie. They want you to believe that their 182 calorie sugar laced cola has the same calorie effect on your weight as 182 calories of broccoli. Don't fall for it.

Personally I have never counted calories and never will. Since I try to eat REAL FOOD *(like Abe Lincoln ate),* I just eat until I am full and then my body always tells me when I have had enough.

This is normal and the way we should all approach eating. All we have to do is listen to our body when we are eating real food.

If you eat real food then your body will be fully satisfied and you will not be hungry for a very long time. But if you eat fake food *(think most anything in a box, bag, can, or frozen),* you will again be hungry soon afterward and then want to find something else to eat.

I find it amusing that every restaurant is going on this *"listing the calories"* kick where all of the menu items are showing how many calories there are.

The typical person then chooses a meal based on the calories and does not realize that the chosen meal is totally laced with sugar and refined carbohydrates. That is why they will never lose the weight that they so desperately want to get rid of.

If it were my choice I would change showing calories on a menu to showing the GLYCEMIC INDEX for each food item on the menu.

Here is the definition for Glycemic Index:

"A system that ranks foods on a scale from 1 to 100 based on their effect on blood-sugar levels."

That way you can then be able to make the wise decision to avoid foods that shoot up your insulin (which is terrible for your health), and then be able to choose foods that will keep your insulin low (which is excellent for your health and weight loss).

Almost every diet program *relies on counting calories* which in my opinion eventually will make your life miserable and promote terrible food choices. People then purchase sugar laced cups of yogurt because the label declares that it only has 100 calories and will fit into their daily calorie counting diet. What they do not understand is that *it is the poor food choices that are keeping them unhealthy.*

In my opinion it is misleading that these TV diet programs tell their audience that they can eat all of the garbage that is flashed on the screen since it is low in calories and will fit into their daily low calorie program.

What they will not tell you is that these types of foods *(pizza, lasagna, ice cream, etc.)* will shoot up your insulin faster than you can say I am being scammed. These are the exact foods that made you gain weight in the first place.

If your insulin is always high not only will you promote various diseases in your body, but your daily energy will be burned using sugar and carbs. It is a terrible choice if you are trying to lose weight.

Keep the insulin low throughout the day and you will then be burning fat as your main energy source (which everyone wishes they could do and is a major key to losing weight). And as a bonus, *good fats allow you to have great energy throughout the day!*

If you are a calorie counter my recommendation is to totally stop doing this and just eat REAL FOOD *(remember 'ol Abe),* and learn to eat the foods that are low on the glycemic index scale (think good fats).

Not only will you feel full for a very long time, but by eating real foods you will begin to see weight melt away.

"Keep the insulin low throughout the day and you will then be burning fat as your energy source (which everyone wishes they could do and is a major key to losing weight). And as a bonus, good fats allow you to have great energy throughout the day!"

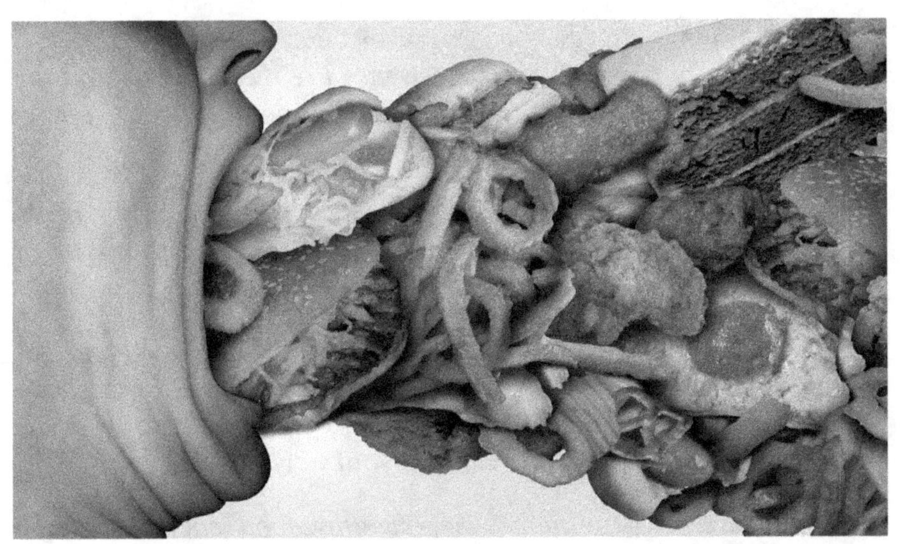

Tip #19
Refined carbohydrate foods are your health enemy

Refined carbohydrates are complex carbs that have had fiber stripped from them leaving simple carbohydrates.

They are then *rapidly digested into our body causing a blood sugar spike*, which is then followed by a sluggish feeling, brain fog, and a rapid crash.

These types of carbs are EMPTY CALORIES and act very similar to the damaging effects of sugar, meaning they make us hate looking into a mirror or getting our picture taken.

Sadly, the Standard American Diet (or SAD Diet) *is blindly followed by the vast majority within our society*. These terrible food choices are also promoted 24/7 on TV commercials which influence the masses to eat a diet made up primarily of refined carbs. These types of foods have very limited nutritional value except to put fat on the body and make us unhealthy.

Trust me when I say that it is very difficult to remove yourself from all of these types of foods since *they are the staple spread for the majority of events, parties, and celebrations that you may attend.*

But here is the important point: *You and you alone are the final deciding factor and will make the ultimate choice of what type of foods will be deposited into your belly.*

I also understand that there will be times when a spread of processed foods is the only viable option to choose from *(been there and done that).* So I do understand that there may be moments when poor food choices are your only option.

My only advice is to *make wise healthy food choices for the majority of your feeding time, especially when you have total control.*

Your body will not only begin to feel lighter with right food choices, but it will also thank you in the future by feeling so much better.

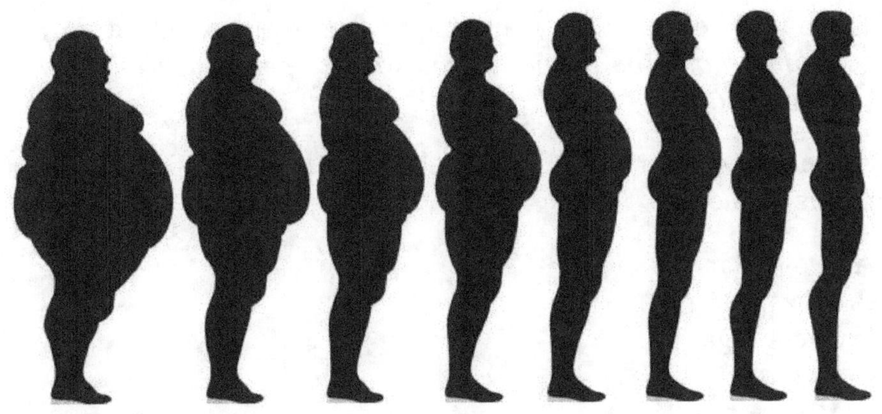

Tip #20
Tired of the dreaded belly fat

Many men and women feel that they have been given a life sentence of having to carry around unwanted belly fat. It can be frustrating and a mystery in figuring out how to get rid of it.

It seems that they have tried everything but still cannot figure out how this belly fat got there in the first place. More importantly, they are frustrated and somewhat clueless in how to eliminate it.

Please listen carefully as I have an easy 1-2 solution that works...

The dreaded overweight belly is nothing more than stored fat from all the years of neglect *stuffing your innocent tummy with sugar and refined carbs.* It is not your belly's fault. The real fault lies in the poor selection of foods that you have deposited into your body for so many years.

So let me get straight to the only answer that will work and you may not like it.

Completely get rid of your longtime friend and comforter know as *sugar* along with all *refined carbs* (think anything in a box), and your belly will eventually get smaller and smaller.

These two items are the main culprit that loves to put fat on our belly *and should be banned if you want to permanently lose that extra weight.*

When I say sugar I am talking about ALL types of crazy sugar names including:

Agave nectar
Brown sugar
Coconut sugar
Corn syrup
Dextrose
Maple syrup
Honey
Sucrose
& on and on and on.

Listen, *sugar is sugar is sugar is sugar* and will always contribute to weight gain.

When I say refined carbs here are a few examples that are bad for your belly:

Most anything in a box, bag, can or frozen

All pastas
All cereals
Bread (including pita breads, etc.)
Pizza (which is mostly bread)
Pastries & Pretzels
Any and all forms of chips (terrible for you)
Cookies, muffins, candies, and all desserts
Frozen dinners
Sauces and most condiments
and yes, your beloved Mac & cheese

Also, totally avoid the below foods as they also convert to sugar in your body and contribute to weight gain:

Potatoes (which is comparable to eating a lump of sugar)
Corn (which is used to fatten cows)
Rice (instantly spikes insulin which is a very bad thing)
Grains (yes, they will eventually make you fat as well)

And remember, going to a gym and doing a billion sit-ups or crunches will not do the trick in getting rid of that tummy. *Losing belly fat only happens in the kitchen.*

My advice would also be to please stop following all of those silly fad diets that eventually fail in the long run.

Simply get rid of sugar and those fattening refined carbohydrate boxed foods and your belly will eventually have to leave.

"Simply get rid of sugar and those fattening refined carbohydrate boxed foods and your belly will eventually have to leave."

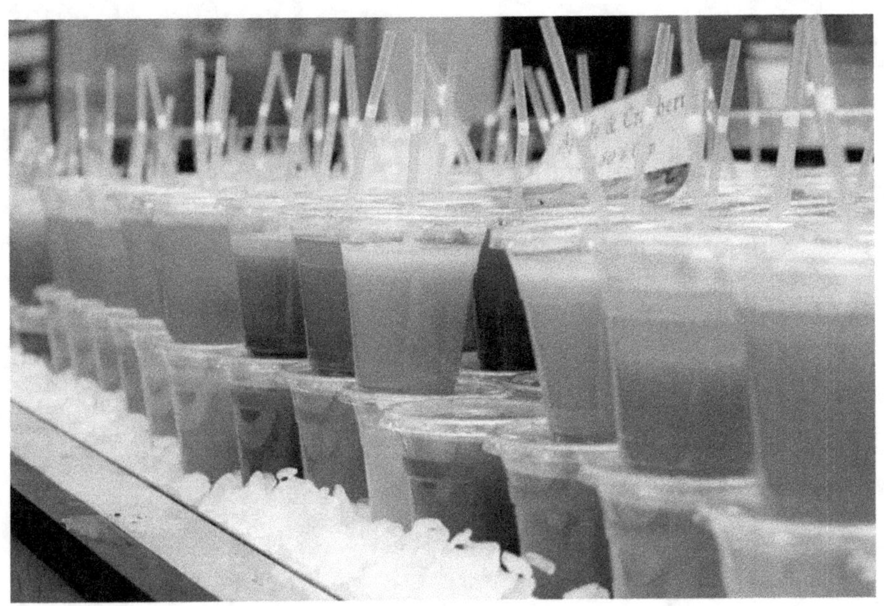

Tip #21
Stop drinking ALL fruit juices

One of the worst drinks to put into your body is any and all types of fruit juices. Whether is it laced with added sugar *or 100% pure juice*, they are all bad for you and will make you unhealthy.

Here are the two reasons why:

1. All of these fruit juices have had the fiber stripped from them which is a terrible ideal for your health. If you must get your orange juice simply choose a regular orange with the fiber instead.

2. Because the juice is seriously concentrated, the minute you gulp it down it instantly spikes your insulin (which is a terrible thing) and whacks your whole body system.

Our bodies are not meant to consume so much concentrated juice (or just call it sugar) all at once. *This amount of concentrated sugar rushing into our system is not a good thing for our health.*

And please stop believing those deceptive TV commercials with the picture perfect family sitting down at breakfast telling you how healthy that their juice is for you.

Nothing could be further from the truth and trust me when I say that you can get your vitamin C from much healthier alternatives.

If you want to improve your health my recommendation is to run far away from any and all types of juices that flood our grocery store aisles. Your health will thank you for it.

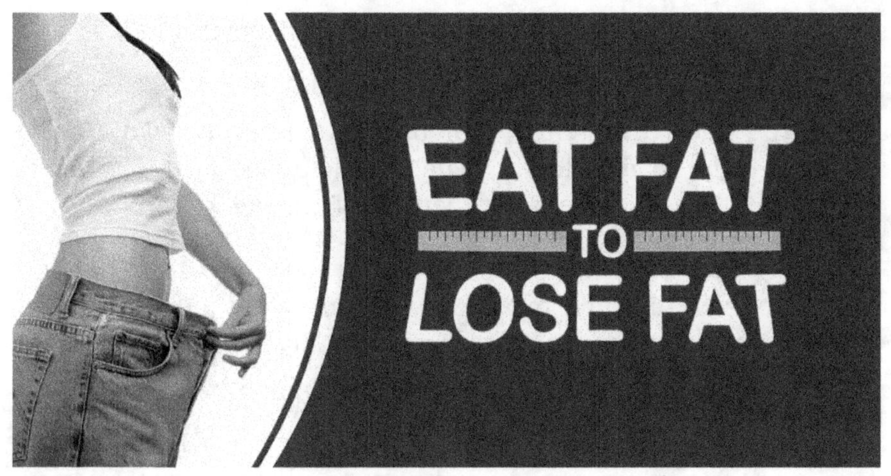

Tip #22
People get fat because they ignore GOOD FATS

I would have to say that the biggest lie perpetrated by our government over the past fifty years is to tell their beloved citizens that all fats are bad for your health. Nothing could be further from the truth. *It is trans fats that we need to avoid.*

We also have this false belief that *"fat makes you fat"* which is absolute ludicrous. Listen, if you want to permanently lose weight then one of the best ways is to make healthy fats a part of your daily diet.

I would also go so far as to say that *good fats can make you lean* and not fat. What will ALWAYS make you fat and sick are trans fats (sorry fried foods, cakes, donuts, margarine, etc.). *There is a world of difference in consuming good fats vs. bad fats.*

I use to be like the majority of our population who avoided all fats like the plague. I was that person who would always only eat white, skinless chicken breast, never touched bacon, always trimmed the fat from my steak, and would always feel guilty and think I was going to become fat after eating an avocado. I was silly and uneducated.

But now I know differently. Our bodies and brains need GOOD FATS in order to function at their complete best. Let me repeat this to all of the naysayers out there again...*GOOD FATS will not and have never made anyone fat.*

Good fats have become my friend and my body and brain keep thanking me for allowing them back into my life. Not only do I feel so much healthier, but my thinking is so much clearer now that I am consuming good fats daily.

Also, good fats fill us up and totally satisfy us for a very long time. Refined carbohydrates *(think boxed & bagged foods)* do the complete opposite. They never truly satisfy, make us gain weight, give us brain fog, and make us hungry again soon after consuming them *(think breads and pastas)*.

Stop believing the lie that all fats are bad for you or make you fat. Just Google it and discover the real reason America has become an obese and unhealthy society ever since fat was vilified back in the 1960's. This then allowed trans fats and refined carbohydrates (processed foods) to become our nation's favorite food sources.

If you still believe the silly premise that "fat makes you fat" then maybe it is time to leave the debunked science of the 1960's and learn the real truth and healthy benefits of making good fats a major part of your daily diet. Your belly and hips will thank you for it.

If you want to lose weight and do your brain and body a big favor then my recommendation is to accept good fats with open arms. You will soon be shopping around for a smaller wardrobe.

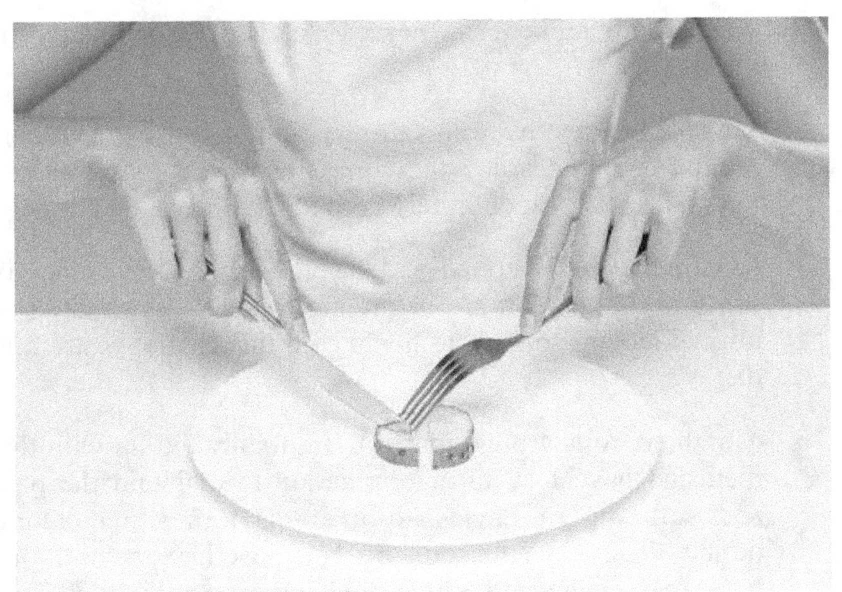

Tip #23
Restricting your calorie intake is a bad idea

The majority of diets all go by the same miserable solution of restricting your daily calorie intake in order to lose those unwanted pounds.

Below is the typical order *of the same old song and dance* for the majority of people who jump head first into following this miserable strategy to lose weight:

1. You are sick and tired of feeling fat.

2. You start the calorie restricting diet with fire in your eyes determined to lose the weight and feel better about yourself.

3. In a short time you begin noticing that your pants are feeling baggier and someone has actually mentioned that

you are looking better. You are on cloud nine and victory is on the way.

4. Three-four months rolls around and so far you've lost around 35 pounds and the compliments are flying at you left and right. You definitely love the moment.

5. Month five rolls around and the fire in your eyes slowly starts to dim as you are beginning to get sick and tired of always feeling somewhat hungry on this calorie restricting diet.

6. Month six rolls around and you are totally fed up with this diet, and have lost all determination to maintain the pain and suffering of having to live this tormenting calorie deficit lifestyle. You soon become just like the millions before you who also became tired and eventually quit.

7. Those 45 pounds that you had lost during the past six months are soon history as you go back to the Standard American Diet (or SAD diet) and begin gaining the weight back with a vengeance.

8. To top it all off, most people will usually gain more weight than they had originally had when they first started the diet.

My advice is to run as fast as possible from any diet that asks you to restrict your daily calories as the majority will eventually fail in the long run. *Please understand that it is the wrong food choices that need to be addressed.*

Understand this important point: The REAL CULPRIT to your weight gain has been *the poor food choices that you have made over the years.*

So what is my recommendation in losing weight? Simply eat REAL FOOD (like Abe Lincoln did). If you could not find a food item in the grocery store that 'ol Abe shopped at, then my recommendation is to keep it out of your kitchen.

Also, divorce from all forms of sugar and refined carbs *(think most foods in a box, bag, can, or frozen),* and you will lose the weight in a healthy and correct manner.

Do this and those extra pounds will eventually fall off permanently because once you begin eating real food and avoid the myriads of terrible factory foods in the grocery stores *(think processed foods),* you will begin to lose weight.

One final thought... I highly recommend Intermittent Fasting everyday as well. It will be a total game changer, totally safe and healthy, and it will give your body rest from constantly stuffing itself. Simply Google *Intermittent Fasting* and educate yourself on this.

"My advice is to run as fast as possible from any diet that asks you to restrict your daily calories as the majority will eventually fail in the long run. Please understand that it is the wrong food choices that need to be addressed."

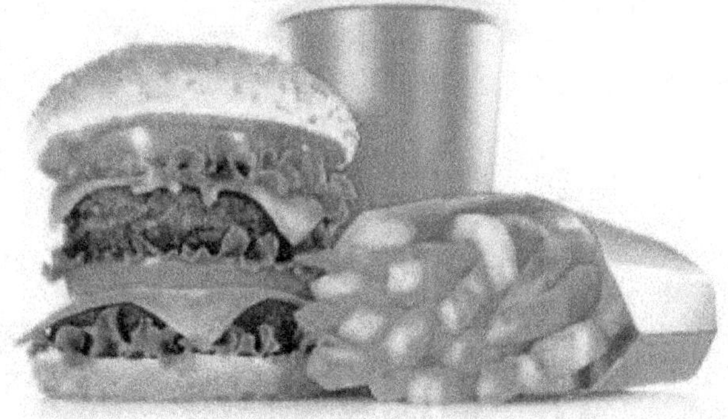

Tip #24
FAKE FOOD or REAL FOOD: Your Choice

When all is said and done and the rubber meets the road in regards to our health, it really does come down to each person individually. Each one of us alone *will ultimately be the final deciding factor* on whether or not we genuinely want to live a healthier lifestyle.

Each one of us also makes the ultimate decision with the food choices that we make for our body, whether good or bad.

For a large majority of our population the choice is to follow the Standard American Diet (SAD Diet) which primarily consists of bad food choices that eventually will play havoc on our overall health.

Here are a few examples of foods that contribute to poor health:

- Refined carbohydrates (most "foods" boxed, bagged, canned or frozen)

- Breads and grains

- Fried foods

- Sugary drinks

- Cereals

- Pastas

- Anything with sugar (to feed our hidden addiction)

One of the major reasons that it is so difficult to leave the SAD Diet is because *these types of foods are everywhere and the hidden sugar in the ingredients makes us want more.*

Food manufacturers are in the business to make a profit and the way that they do this is to make their processed foods taste as yummy as possible. We need to also remember that company profits *will always trump the future overall health of a customer.*

Their deceptive marketing and packaging may fool the customer into thinking that the boxed product is healthy, but please be aware that the vast majority of anything in a box is detrimental to your overall health.

My recommendation is to avoid as much as possible the majority of these types of manufactured boxed, bagged, canned, or frozen foods that fill up the aisles at your friendly local grocery store. As said earlier, it is all about profits, period.

Go online and educate yourself on how to make better food choices by learning to eat real food instead of these manufactured foods that were created in a basement factory.

In the end, it will be you and you alone who will make the final decision in the types of foods that your body will be fed. Learn to make wise choices *and your health will thank you for it.*

"For a large majority of our population the choice is to follow the Standard American Diet (SAD Diet) which primarily consists of bad food choices that eventually will play havoc on our overall health."

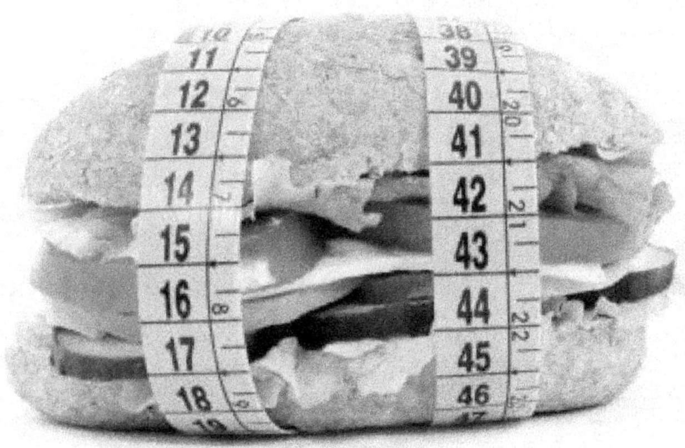

Tip #25
Breads and bagels bring the bulge

No matter how you slice it all forms of store breads put on the weight. Don't believe anyone who says otherwise as breads convert to sugar once digested, raise our insulin, and then stores that yucky stuff called fat on our innocent bodies.

Quick crazy fact: A slice of whole wheat bread raises our insulin *(a really bad thing)* faster than a yummy Snickers bar.

The reason bread is so popular is that it is very cheap and a very profitable commodity for every restaurant and fast food joint on the planet. Just ask Subway or Jimmy Johns.

I hate to say this but *all of the breads* at our beloved Panera Bread will expand our waistline. It does not matter who is serving it as all bought breads will put weight on us. The same goes for all of those cracker boxes in the grocery aisle.

Even our government has been telling us for decades that we need our daily supply of good old bread. And didn't even Jesus tell us that man shall not live by bread alone, but by every word that proceeds out of the mouth of God.

But trust me when I say that the bread being consumed today is a totally different beast than centuries prior to now. And if you are attempting to lose the bulge and eat bread every day, you might as well eat snicker bars instead.

It just seems so un-American to even make a statement that bread is not good for you. Just look at our trusted US food pyramid and guess who is smack right in the middle at the very bottom telling uninformed citizens that bread needs to be consumed every day.

When I say bread I am talking about more than all of those bread loaves in your grocery store aisle. It comes in all shapes and sizes. It is that tasty chewy flat round bottom holding up the toppings on your pizza as well as those pretty rolls in that nice wicker basket on that fancy restaurant table.

Two great books to learn more about the ill effects of making bread a daily staple in your life is *Grain Brain* by David Perlmutter and *Wheat Belly* by William Davis as they both do an excellent job at exposing the danger of today's bread.

If you are serious about getting rid of that bulge that has been bothering you for years, I would first and foremost recommend making bread a thing of the past.

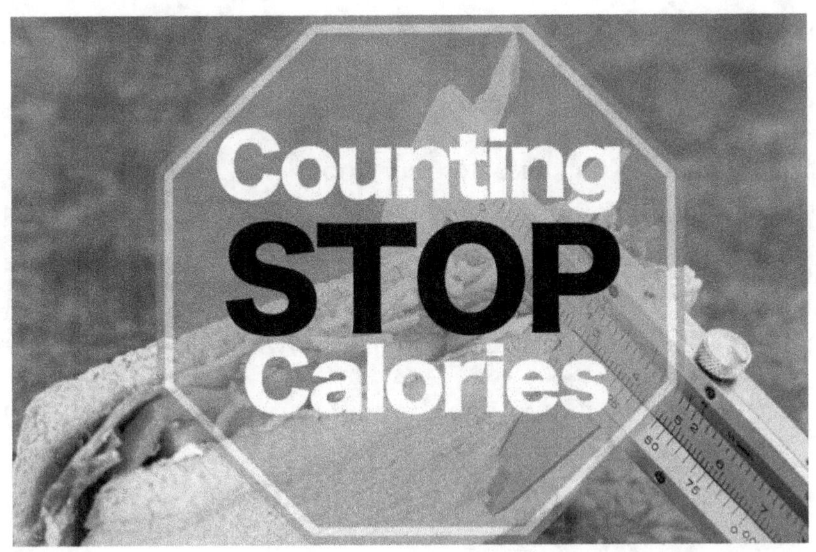

Tip #26
STOP counting calories to lose weight

It always boggles my brain when I hear that someone is counting every jot and tittle in an attempt to lose weight.

One word of advice: *Counting calories eventually fails and will make your life miserable after the motivation wears off.*

Instead of counting calories let me give you a more novel idea that works much better and keeps your belly happy and satisfied.

Here it is:

Just eat REAL FOODS *(just like our 'ol friend Abe Lincoln did)* and divorce all forms of sugar and refined carbohydrates (processed foods). Forget about silly calorie counting and simply stop eating all of those *made in a factory processed foods* that more than likely made you overweight in the first place

The culprit is the *poor food choices* made over the years and nothing more. Your body hates these cheap processed foods and has rebelled by storing fat on your hips and belly.

Simply change your diet to real foods and your weight will eventually begin to drop to where it should be.

Trust me when I say that your body will begin to melt away that unwanted fat. The answer has never been found in calorie counting. *The real answer is found in removing bad food from your life.*

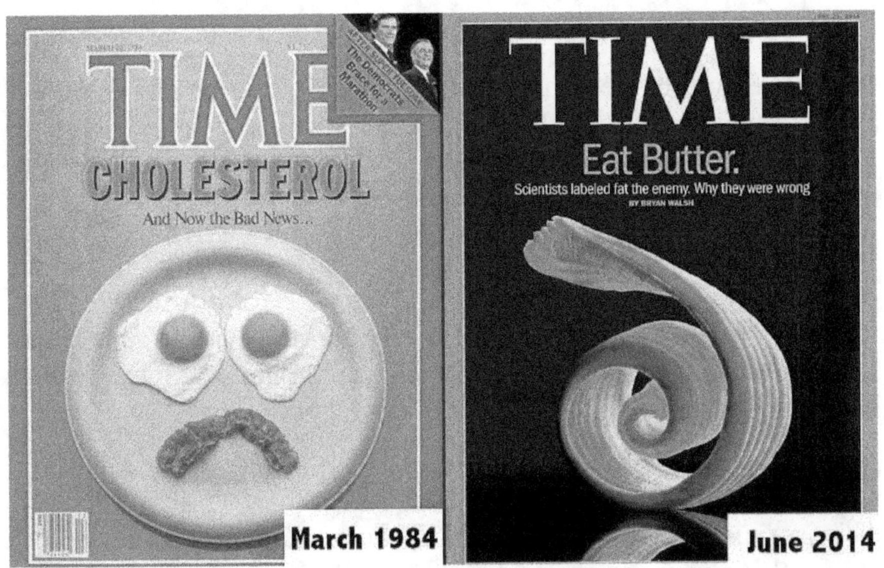

Tip #27
The 3 major benefits of eating GOOD FATS

Our bodies crave good fats and the vilifying of fats over the past 50 years has to go down as one of the saddest blips in US history for America's health. We as a nation have been brainwashed into believing that all fats are our enemy. Trans fats are the real enemy.

I personally believe that this wrong advice has created a train wreck on the overall health of Americans. It is hard to believe that so many people even today are still swallowing this old wives' tale hook, line and sinker.

If you are one of those still living in the 1960's please reeducate yourself by going to Google and catch up to the truth that our bodies need good fats.

Here are my three personal favorite benefits of eating GOOD FATS everyday:

#1 YOUR BODY NEEDS GOOD FATS

Stop believing the lie that good fats will clog you up and give you a heart attack or bad cholesterol. Better yet, just type into Google "The Great Cholesterol Myth" and you will soon discover that the majority of what we have believed about cholesterol is wrong.

We as humans have been eating fats for thousands of years and all of a sudden we have been told that all fats are bad for us. We have followed this silly advice and replaced good fats with terrible sugar laced products, processed foods, and damaging trans fats which have resulted in an unhealthy and overweight society.

#2 GOOD FATS KEEP YOUR INSULIN LOW

This is a major point and I would encourage anyone to learn to eat foods that keep your insulin low. When our insulin is low throughout the day we are then allowed to burn fat as our main energy source *(which everyone wishes that they could do).*

But when our insulin is consistently high *(due to the Standard American Diet or SAD Diet),* we spend our days burning sugar and carbs as our main energy source and wonder why we cannot lose that fat around our belly and hips.

On a side note, I find it amusing that people will eat something like a banana (an insulin spiker) before working out without realizing that for the next few hours they will only be burning sugar and carbs instead of fat that they so desperately want to lose.

#3 GOOD FATS MAKE US FEEL FULLER FOR A LONGER TIME

This is my personal favorite as I soon discovered early on that eating good fats totally makes me feel full for a very, very long time. Trust me when I say that those nice juicy steaks that I make on the grill keep me satisfied for hours upon hours.

You will not be hungry for a long time which will also allow weight to start falling off of your body.

Good fats will not make a person fat. It is just the opposite as eating good fats allows our body to then burn fat (due to a low insulin level) and thus creates a great environment for weight loss.

The reason most people are always hungry is simply because their daily diets are made up primarily of refined carbohydrates (food in a box) which never truly makes us satisfied, but ends up giving us a craving for more of these types of processed foods.

My advice to anyone is to include a healthy amount of good fats into your daily diet and watch your overall health improve.

"If you are one of those still living in the 1960's please reeducate yourself by going to Google and catch up to the truth that our bodies need good fats."

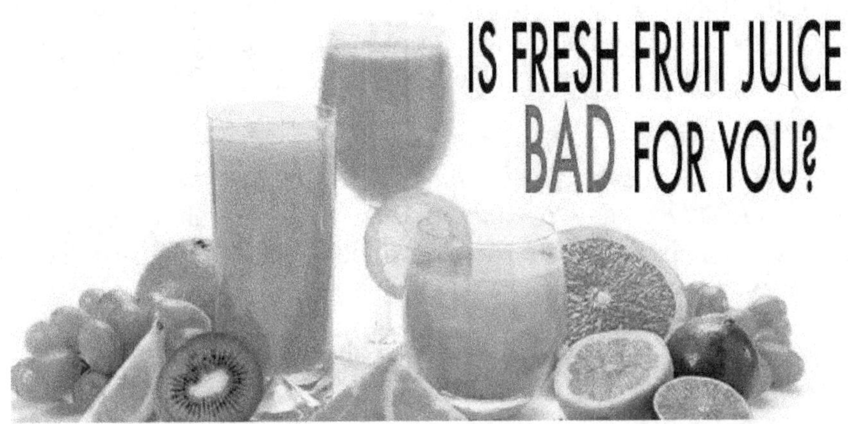

Tip #28
Run far, far away from juice bars

Walk into any mall and you are sure to find a juice bar with the intention of making potential customers believe that their juice drinks are the healthiest product on the planet.

Nothing could be further from the truth. My advice is to save your five bucks and run as fast as you can from these high insulin pumping drinks.

This also includes bottles that populate the shelves at your friendly grocery store. And no, they are not healthy for you at all.

These sugar concentrated products go by many names such as Jamba Juice, Naked Fruit, Smoothie King, Clean Juice, Mr. Smoothie, and on and on and on.

If you want to stay unhealthy, instantly spike your insulin level, and feel sluggish for a few hours after your last sip from a straw, then by all means enjoy the ride.

So what is my problem with these juice bars that look so healthy on the outside, especially since they promote that their smoothies are the healthiest drink on the planet? Even all of their pictures on the wall show happy and healthy looking people sipping away on one of their sugar laced smoothies. How can this stuff really be bad for you?

Here is my answer: *All of these drinks are HIGHLY CONCENTRATED fructose drinks* that instantly shoot up your insulin (which is a terrible thing), which then stores all of these calories as fat on your body.

Our bodies also go into a quiet state of shock as *we simply are not designed to consume such a large amount of this highly concentrated sugary stuff.*

First of all they add fruit juice (terrible for your body) to your five dollar drink followed by whatever fruit you want. You need to understand that the amount of sugar (fructose) in this drink is really bad for your body.

Remember, *the more sugar you eat, the more fat you will store.* More specifically, too much sugar, even from the fructose found in these fruit drinks, can lead to a buildup of that visceral belly fat that has been linked to type 2 diabetes.

I scratch my head that so many people out there are being deceived by these "healthy" juice drinks and smoothies, but do not realize that *the amount of sugar in these drinks are detrimental to any person's health.*

My advice is to avoid any and all of these fruit drinks. I commend you for attempting to want to be healthier, but going to a juice bar is not the way to go.

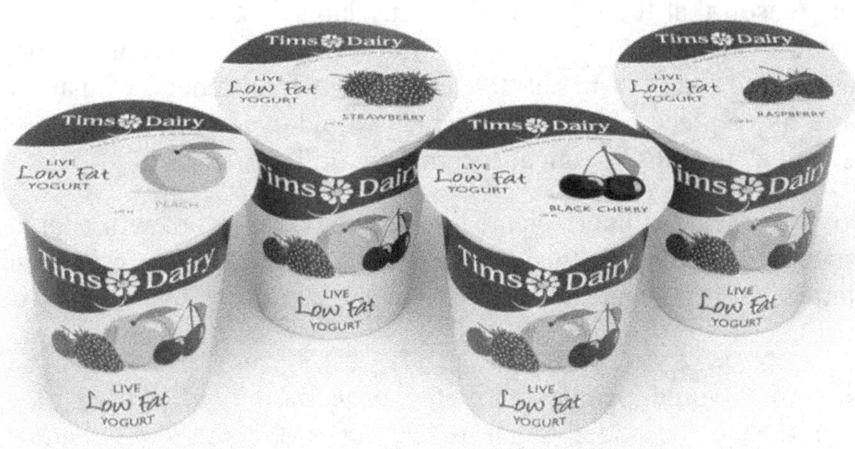

Tip #29
Avoid anything that says "low fat" or "no fat"

A few years back every food company on the planet began labeling their food products with the words "low fat" or "no fat" in a sneaky attempt to not only sell more products, but also give the customer a false impression that the food item must be healthy.

America soon bought into this low/no fat kick and it soon appeared that every other product on the grocery shelves was proudly telling the world that their product did not have that evil fat in it.

When fat was officially vilified over 50 years ago as the scapegoat to every health problem under the sun, this declaration soon promoted sugar and refined carbs as the good guys.

Since all fats now became the enemy of the state, our food laboratory scientists in white coats came up with a brilliant food idea… take the fat out of a food product and replace it with highly addictive sugar and refined carbohydrates.

The reason that the big food company lab scientists with the thick glasses and bad breath made the switch was because they discovered that taking natural fat out of a food tended to make it taste like a piece of cardboard which would eventually effect sales as well as the CEO's annual $56 million dollar salary.

So with their brilliant scientist minds they came up with a great strategy by replacing this evil fat *with highly addictive sugar* and started calling sugars by different names in order to confuse the customer.

Not only would people enjoy the taste more, *but getting them addictive* to the added sugar would produce more sales. I mean seriously, who can eat just one graham cracker?

The bottom line is this: *Stop being afraid of the good fats found naturally in foods.* GOOD FATS are your friends.

Whenever our caring scientists take out the fat in any product they are replacing it with either sugar, processed carbs, or something that you cannot pronounce, which of course is really bad for your health and waistline.

My advice is to throw away anything in your kitchen with the silly label proudly declaring that it is "low fat" or "no fat". More than likely the product has been laced with the fat producing white stuff called sugar (think low/no fat yogurt).

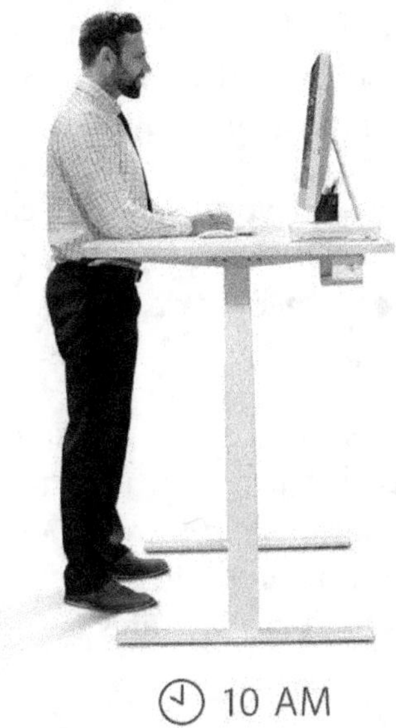

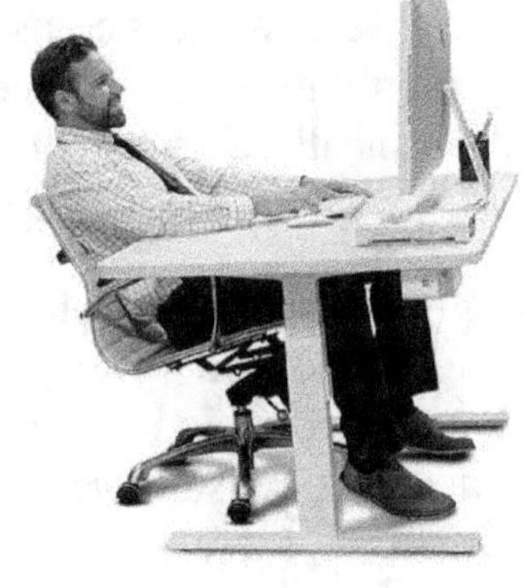

Tip #30
Sitting eight hours a day is terrible for you

I would have to say that the absolute worst consequences in our age of computers is that the majority in our workforce sits at a desk all day as they slowly put on weight staring at a screen while eating their Egg McMuffin and fat producing blueberry muffin.

It has been declared that sitting is the new smoking and is said to be comparable to smoking a pack of cigarettes every day. Either way, we all agree that sitting for long periods of time is detrimental to anyone's health.

Plain and simple, we as humans *were not meant to sit all day* and look at a computer (or TV for that manner). But in today's technology world the vast majority of workers are sitting for eight or more hours a day trying to earn a paycheck.

Here is my suggestion to this terrible dilemma: Buy a stand up desk to work at. Either ask your company if they offer an option to provide a stand up desk, and if not then purchase one yourself.

It will be well worth the cash forked over and your overall health will seriously improve. As mentioned earlier, we as humans are not meant to sit all day. *Just the simple act of standing at a desk will do wonders for your overall health.*

One of my best personal health moves was purchasing a stand up desk and cannot tell you what a difference it has made. Pictured is the model I ordered (from www.autonomous.ai) and they seriously have a very reasonable price when compared to the other companies out there. You can also easily adjust the stand up desk to any height with a push of a button.

Please do yourself and your health a giant favor and purchase a stand up desk ASAP. You will soon see the different in how you feel.

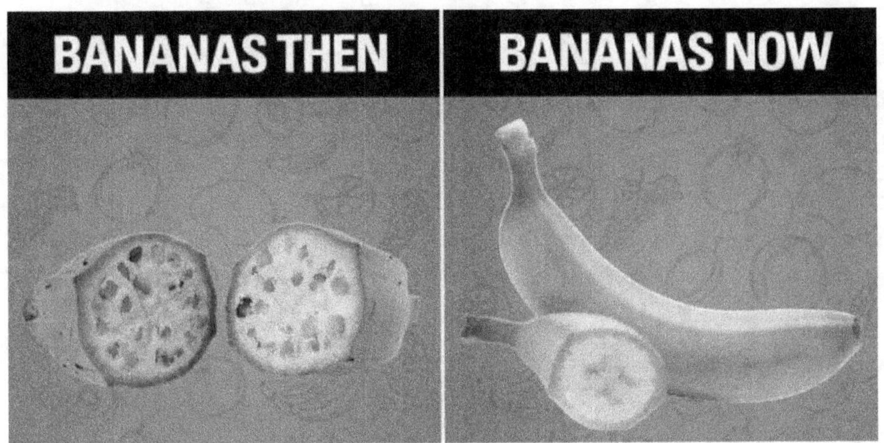

Tip #31
Here is my take on fruit

A question that often arises is what are my views on fruits and are they good for us? A great question and here is my personal feelings about the majority of fruits out there.

First off, most fruits today have been modified from their original origin. Simply Google what fruits use to look like and you will clearly see that many of today's fruits are a totally different breed.

Second, fruit is loaded with fructose (sugar) and instantly raises your insulin which is a bad thing. The lesser-known fact is that fructose, or fruit sugars, acts just like any other sugar when it comes to how your body reacts.

All sugars (whether coming from a banana or snickers bar) raise your insulin which then makes you burn sugar and carbs as an energy source instead of burning your fat as energy (which everyone wishes they could do).

Remember, *the more sugar you eat, the more fat your body will want to store.* Specifically, too much sugar, even from the fructose found in fruits, can lead to maintaining a high insulin level.

As for myself, I personally keep fruit to a minimum since my goal is to keep my insulin level as low as possible throughout the day. I also pick out fruits that are low on the glycemic index (meaning low sugar). Examples are berries such as blue berries and black berries.

So what is my recommendation? Keep fruits to a minimum in order to keep your insulin low. I also would recommend totally avoiding any fruit juices as well. If you want orange juice it is much better to simply eat an orange as you will at least get the fiber in the fruit.

Sure a banana may be better than a snickers bar, but remember that both will raise your insulin. Keep your insulin low and your health will improve.

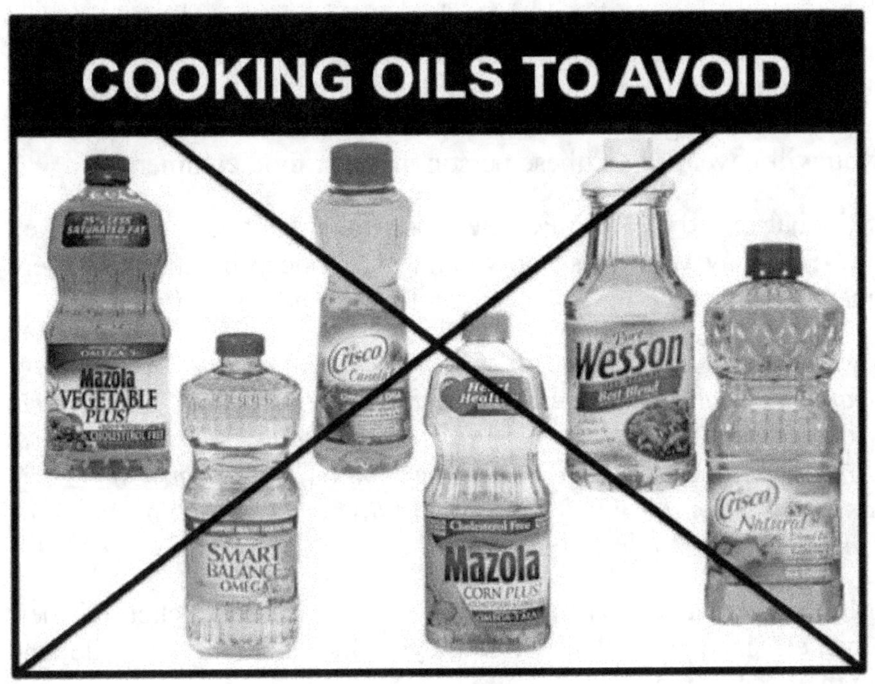

Tip #32
KFC, Popeyes, and other grease joints

We live in a day and age where cheap food is pedaled at every other street corner with the simple convenience of just talking into an outdoor menu box and getting a bag of food through a small window from a bored teenager in no time flat.

We love the convenience but hate the weight gain that is always included with the bag when visiting any of these fat, I mean fast food joints. If only we could have the convenience without the eventual price tag of putting on more weight.

Not to gross anyone out, but the majority of us really do not know exactly what we are eating and neither do we care. All we know is that it is finger lickin' good!

That golden pile of chicken looks mighty good on the TV commercial. Have you also ever noticed that everyone who is in the commercial looks healthy and lean while they smile and munch away on their greasy chicken leg? Trust me also when I say that you will never see an obese person in a fast food commercial.

So what exactly does KFC use to fry their famous recipe chicken in? You may want to sit down and take a deep breath since there may be some who may want to faint after reading what they use:

"KFC products are fried in oil which may contain the following: Canola Oil and Hydrogenated Soybean Oil with TBHQ and Citric Acid Added to Protect Flavor, Dimethylpolysiloxane, an Antifoaming Agent Added OR Low Linolenic Soybean Oil, TBHQ and Citric Acid Added to Protect Flavor, Dimethylpolysiloxane, and an Antifoaming Agent Added."

Makes me want to run out and grab a whole bucket of their chicken since now I know that they include Dimethylpolysiloxane in their secret recipe at no extra charge.

Let me get straight to the point concerning all of the fried food menu items at ANY given restaurant, and that is that *they are terrible for your health.*

It does not matter if it is a fried appetizer at Chilis, seasoned French fries at Red Robin, a morning hash brown from McDonald's, or Friday night fish and chips at your favorite hole in the wall, all of these fried foods are another major reason why so many people are unhealthy and carrying extra weight.

Restaurants all use FAKE and unhealthy cooking oils mixed with who knows what whenever a food is deep fried. *All of these cooking oils are detrimental for your health* and should be avoided like the black plague.

If you absolutely must fry then use olive oil or coconut oil. Both are excellent choices with some serious great health benefits. Now if only every restaurant did the same.

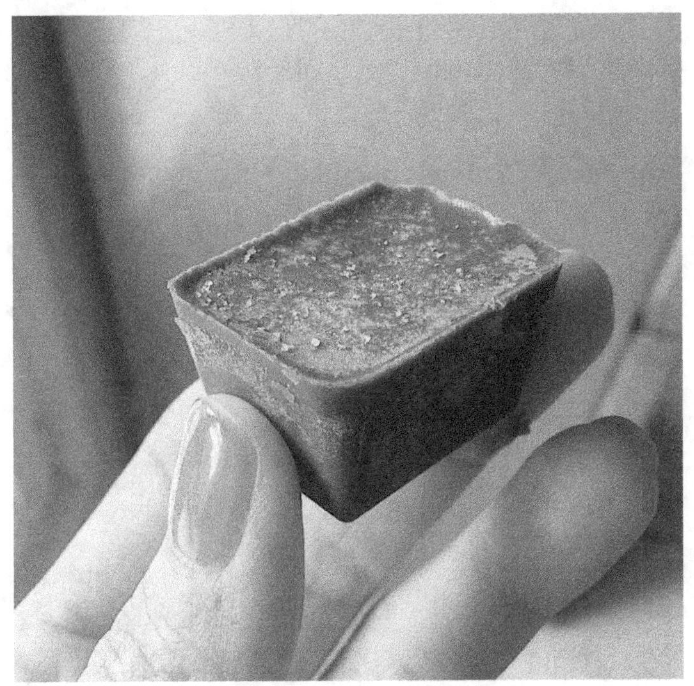

Tip #33
Satisfy your sweet tooth with FAT BOMBS

Of all the short health articles that I have written this is going to be my absolute favorite simply because I am about to share with you a little secret that I always eat after a home meal and totally satisfies my sweet tooth day in and day out.

It is my ultimate favorite and basically only dessert that never gets old. And here is the real kicker...*it is totally healthy for me and will not put an ounce of fat on a person like all of those sugar laced desserts do.* It tastes amazing and honestly do not know how I could have lived without them.

So what is this "dessert" that I am putting on a pedestal? They are simply called Fat Bombs and once you try them you will NEVER want to go back to any of the dozens of sugar laced desserts that not only expand your belly, but make you feel lethargic for two hours after consuming them.

Fat bombs have 4 ingredients and that's it. Here is the recipe:

1 cup of melted coconut oil (love this stuff)
2 tbsp. of cocoa powder
1 tsp. of stevia (I order the plant powder online so no chemicals involved)
Splash of vanilla

*Optional: slivered almonds and 100% straight coconut flakes

1. Mix the top four ingredients in a pouring bowl.

2. Get 1-2 empty ice cube trays and fill the bottom with the optional slivered almonds and/or coconut flakes.

3. Now simply pour the liquid coconut oil mix into each tray cube and then put them in the freezer for 30 minutes.

4. From there simply pop the frozen Fat Bombs out of the tray and then always keep them in the freezer in a zip lock bag.

Once you are ready to eat these beautiful and healthy desserts put a couple of frozen Fat Bombs in a bowl with a scoop of 100% natural peanut butter to dip into. You will think you are eating a delicious peanut butter cup.

As a final note, I love to add blue berries or black berries in the bowl as an extra treat as well. Just make sure to eat Fat Bombs when they are frozen as in my opinion they taste the best that way.

If you are serious about losing weight but are fighting a sweet tooth, my recommendation is to fall in love with Fat Bombs. You will never want to return to those unhealthy fat producing desserts after you've had one of these!

Tip #34
How long does it take is the wrong question to ask

When I am approached about learning to eat healthy foods the inevitable question eventually comes up:

"How long will it take to lose the weight?"

Let me answer this question in the kindest way possible.

We are not talking about a certain time frame or a silly gimmick in an attempt to lose weight. What we are talking about is a complete eating lifestyle change *and nothing less.*

It is all about doing a 180 degree turn in leaving your past poor food choices completely. If you want to succeed for life in maintaining a healthy weight *it means never going back to the terrible diet that made you gain weight in the first place.*

So many people spend their whole lives wandering from one silly diet to the next in a desperate attempt to find that miracle diet or pill that will shed the weight off permanently. But I've said this many times and will repeat it again:

"Calorie restrictive diets do not and have never worked in the long run. Only a complete separation from your old food choices (think food in a box) is the final solution to healthy and permanent weight loss."

The major reason that people fail diets is simply because they eventually revert back to the comforting Standard American Diet (or SAD Diet) which continues to produce a nation of obese people.

Please stop putting a time limit on when the weight will come off. It took you years (sometimes decades) to pack the weight on. Eat REAL FOODS and the weight will come off in a healthy and timely manner.

My advice is to give it time and your body will naturally take care of itself by rewarding you with weight loss as you divorce all types of sugar and refine carbohydrates from your diet.

I would also recommend not thinking that changing to a better eating habit is a diet you are trying. Instead, look at it *as a total lifestyle change* from eating terrible foods to eating the food that we were intended to eat, and that is real foods.

Do this, allow time, and trust me when I say that your body will reward you by letting go of the weight that you so desperately would like to lose.

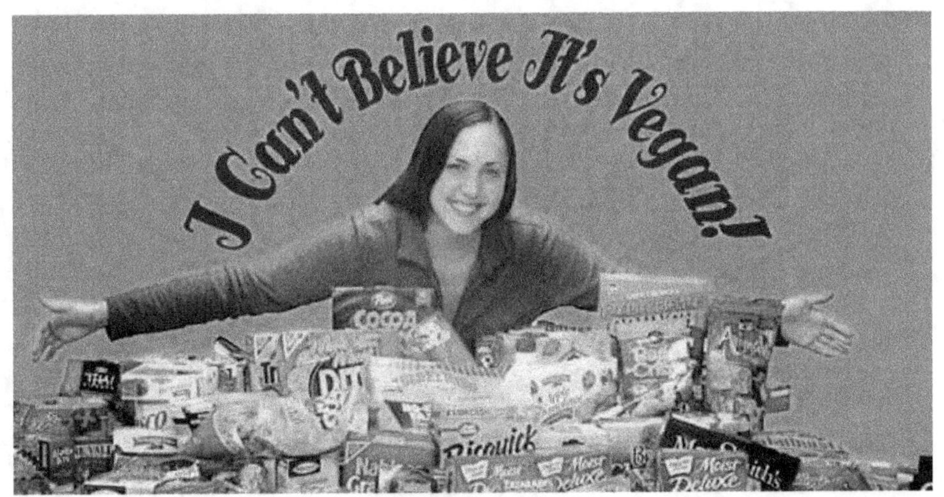

Tip #35
Here are my thoughts on the vegetarian lifestyle

I respect anyone who wants to dive into the vegetarian lifestyle, whether it is to eat better, live healthier, or simply for a moral issue. And I am also aware that there are different levels within the framework of living a vegetarian lifestyle.

But avoiding either animal products or meats (especially with the hormones being used) does not necessarily make us automatically healthy.

I get it as I also have watched the sad documentaries on farms and how animals are being treated, and from a moral standpoint I have absolutely no problem with a person's personal conviction in becoming a vegetarian on these grounds alone.

But this is not what the article is about. What I want to focus on is exactly how healthy is the vegetarian lifestyle as a whole.

And here is where I scratch my head and need to address just how healthy this eating lifestyle really is. For the vegetarian, eating either all animal products or simply meat has been banished from their life. And that is fine with me.

But I have also noticed that for so many following this chosen lifestyle they continue to eat poorly by consistently eating sugar and processed foods as a main stable in their diet.

Simply because we decide to stop eating meat does not equate to automatically becoming a healthier person. Sure you do not have to deal with the hormones being pumped into these poor animals (unless they are totally free from these and grass fed), but what about all of the refined carbs (think food in a box) that may be part of your diet?

The bottom line is that we need to simply stay away from sugar and processed foods as this is the real culprit to our health crisis in America. If a person has a conviction to avoid meat then it is his or her choice alone to make that decision. But becoming truly healthy will not work if we continue to eat all of these refined carbs.

Believing that we automatically become healthy due to a vegetarian lifestyle is just not true if we are also including boxed, bagged, canned or frozen foods as part of our diet (think pastas, breads, pancakes, bagels, cereals, and everything in between).

No matter what eating lifestyle you decide to follow, every expert in the field of nutrition agrees that sugar and processed foods are terrible for our health and should be avoided.

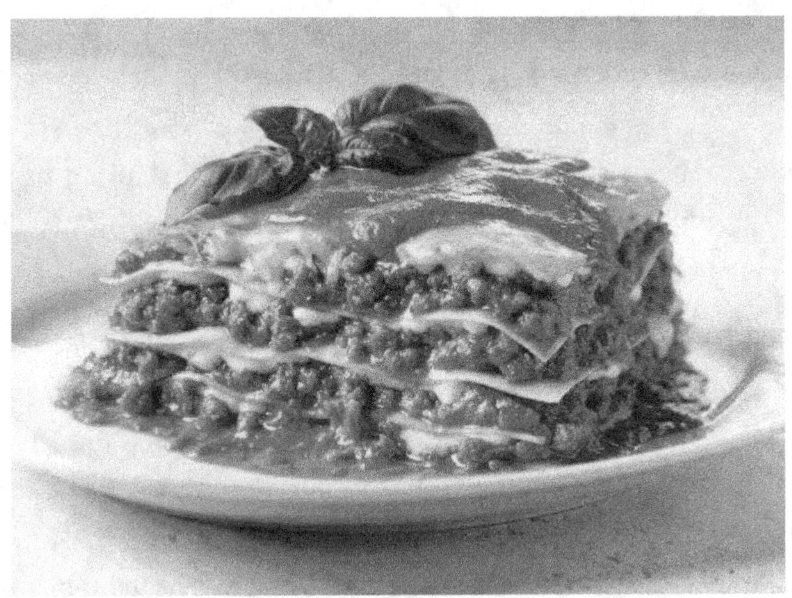

Tip #36
Dealing with Aunt Betty and her famous lasagna dish

So let's say that you are totally committed to changing your lifestyle to healthy eating and are sold on the fact that from this day forward you are going to just eat REAL FOOD *(similar to what ol' Abe Lincoln would have eaten)*.

But what about those sticky moments when your Aunt Betty invites you and the family over for her world famous lasagna dish? What in the world do you do now without upsetting Aunt Betty and the dish that has gone down within the family circle as legendary?

Trust me when I say that there will always be moments like this as long as we have our feet planted on this earth. How in the world do we handle these times in our life?

My advice is to bite the bullet and shove the lasagna down your esophagus in order not to upset the apple cart and have people whispering.

I believe above all else conveying love takes first place over a carb-on-steroids dish any day of the year.

I always like to say that we can control about 95% of the food that goes down the hatch and the other 5% food control needs to be reserved for those moments when Aunt Betty pinches our cheek and tells us to eat more.

Even though you are going to go through brain fog for a few hours after punishing your body with this instant insulin rush dish, it will be worth the satisfaction that Aunt Betty has in feeding you.

Personally, I really do not like being "that guy" at the table who takes a rain check on the delicious insulin spiking rolls being passed around and really do try to enjoy the thick carb-rich pizza when that is the only option.

So remember that there will be those brief moments in life when you may have to bend like the willow tree, and as they say in the food world, when in Rome, carbonate like the Romans!

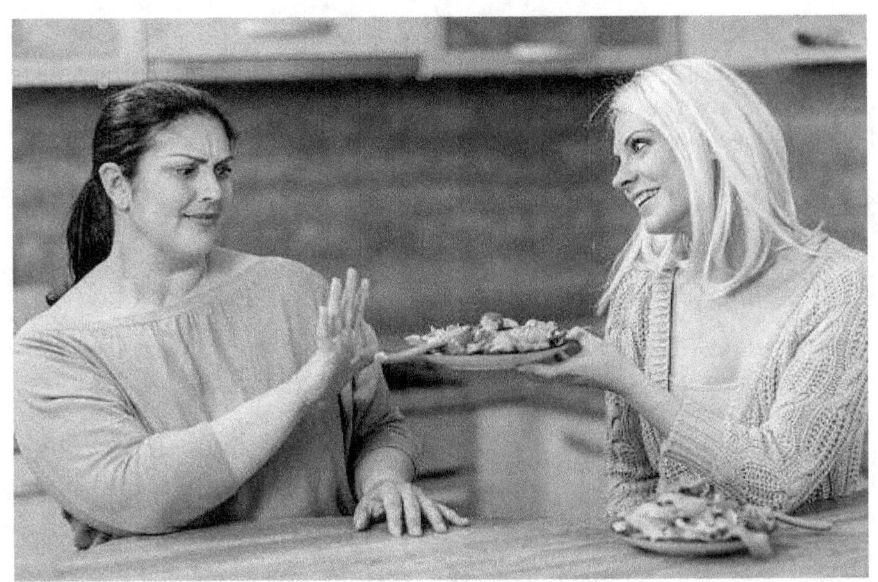

Tip #37
When family members are not on board

I have been asked this question in regards to how to handle other family members (like a spouse) who is addicted to the Standard American Diet (or SAD Diet) and has no intention of ever leaving his or her food in a box diet. What now?

Here is my immediate response to anyone who needs an answer to this dilemma. My answer is short and sweet:

"Never, ever force ANYONE to change their food habits as it is their complete right to eat anyway they want to eat. It is their belly and they should be allowed to fill it up with anything they want."

I believe that no person has a right to dictate what another person chooses to eat. Of course we all want our loved ones to eat REAL FOOD in order to be healthy. *But it is not our right to tell them what to eat.*

I have learned that when it comes to the topic of food we need to walk with caution. For many people food is a sacred matter and to even bring up the topic of eating healthier can instantly become a bee in the bonnet.

So what is my advice when your spouse thinks that you have lost your mind and are just going through another new silly diet phrase?

My advice is to simply stay true to your own conviction in eating real food and weeding out sugar and processed foods.

It may take some time, but trust me when I say that you will begin to feel better, look more attractive, and grow a sharper mind now that you have rid this toxin known as sugar out of your system.

The new you that will eventually emerge will be noticed by both family and friends and you won't have to say a word as they begin asking you the secret to your newfound health.

Now you have earned the right to speak to listening ears.

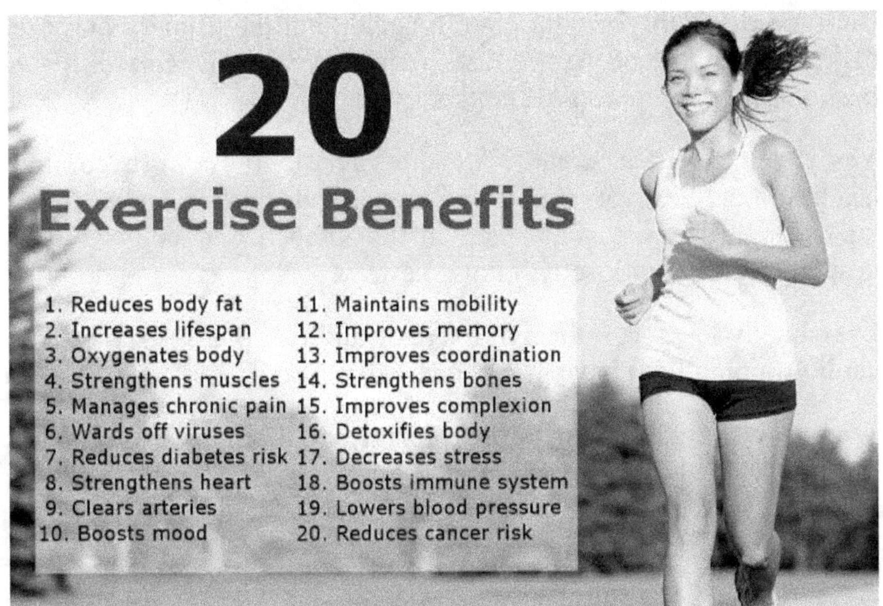

Tip #38
The clear benefits of exercise

There are two primary forms of exercise that offer great benefits for those who are disciplined to make it part of their life. Here are the main two types of exercise:

1. *Resistance Training*
   Resistance training is a form of exercise that improves muscular strength and endurance. Whether it is using weights, bands, or your own body weight, the overall purpose is to strengthen and tone your muscular system.

2. *Cardio Training*
   Cardio training is any exercise that raises your heart rate. Whether it is walking, running, or using a wide variety of aerobic movements, the overall purpose is to strengthen your cardiovascular system.

Both are excellent for your overall health, but the primary purpose of each should not be to lose weight *since this can only be accomplished by radically changing your diet.*

Yes, exercise is a great start on your journey in becoming healthier, and yes, you may lose a few pounds huffing and puffing, but without a smart game plan in the kitchen that belly you so desperately want to lose will not go away.

I personally love each form of exercise and feel that resistance and cardio training both have great benefits.

When I was training for both ironman competitions my primary focus was targeted toward cardio training and very little on resistance training since the 140 mile day called for my cardio system to get me through the event.

It was extreme and I will admit that events like these call for a certain personality (crazy being one of them). But when it comes to cardio training my recommendation is to keep it much simpler.

Whether it is walking around the neighborhood, doing a short 1-3 mile jog, or joining an aerobics class, the goal is to build your endurance.

I also highly recommend resistance training for everyone. Whether it is using your body weight (pushups for example), using strength bands, or lifting weights at home or in the gym, the benefits are outstanding.

The main purpose of resistance training is to strengthen your muscular system which brings about a more toned body and makes it much easier to perform daily tasks like moving or lifting.

I highly recommend getting into the habit of making exercise a part of your life since *the benefits will always outweigh the time that you have spent in the gym.*

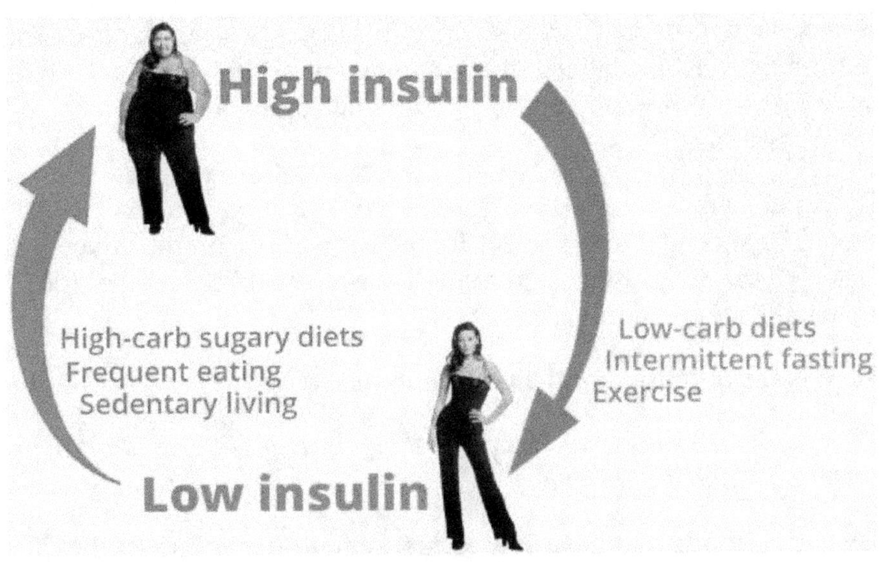

Tip #39
Intermittent Fasting allows your body to burn fat longer

I am simply amazed that very few people understand the importance of our insulin level in regards to how it affects weight gain or weight loss.

Here is what you need to know:

When your daily diet consists of foods that instantly spike your insulin level (think sugars and refined carbs), you go into a state of burning sugar and carbs as your main energy source instead of using body fat as your primary energy source *(which we all want to do)*.

Here is an example... you wake up in the morning and think you are eating healthy by munching on a banana and bagel with orange juice as a chaser.

But what you do not understand is that these three products are absolutely terrible choices for losing weight as they instantly spike your insulin level due to the high amount of sugar in all three of these breakfast items.

If you are going to eat breakfast *(which I do not recommend),* it would be much better to select foods that are low on the Glycemic Index. This way your insulin will stay low because the foods selected have a low sugar index.

Here is the definition of the Glycemic Index:

"A system that ranks foods on a scale from 1 to 100 based on their effect on blood-sugar levels."

By eating foods that have low sugar content, we are now allowing our bodies to burn its own fat as an energy source.

Here is the math:

Maintain low insulin = Burn fat = Lose weight
Maintain high insulin = Burn sugar/carbs = Keep or gain weight

This is one major reason that I love Intermittent Fasting which simply is skipping breakfast and not eating until at least noon. That way you are allowing your body up to 16 hours to fast *and prolong a "fat burning mode" body state.*

When we fast (even in our sleep) our insulin level eventually drops and we are then able to burn fat. But the mistake that the majority of Americans make is that they wake up in a healthy low insulin state *and right away grab an unhealthy high sugar content breakfast that instantly shoots their insulin back up.*

Whenever I see an obese person my first thought is that their insulin level is consistently high. Since they never give their body rest from foods that produce high insulin, they spend their day burning sugars and carbs as their primary energy source.

My simple advice would be to *learn to eat REAL FOODS which consistently keep our insulin low throughout the day*, resulting in burning fat as our primary energy source.

My recommendation is to learn to keep your insulin low by Intermittent Fasting as well as selecting foods that are low on the Glycemic index.

If you want to lose weight and feel better then you will need to learn to avoid foods that spike up your insulin *(think sugar and processed foods)*.

"If you want to lose weight and feel better then you will need to learn to avoid foods that spike up your insulin (think sugar and processed foods)."

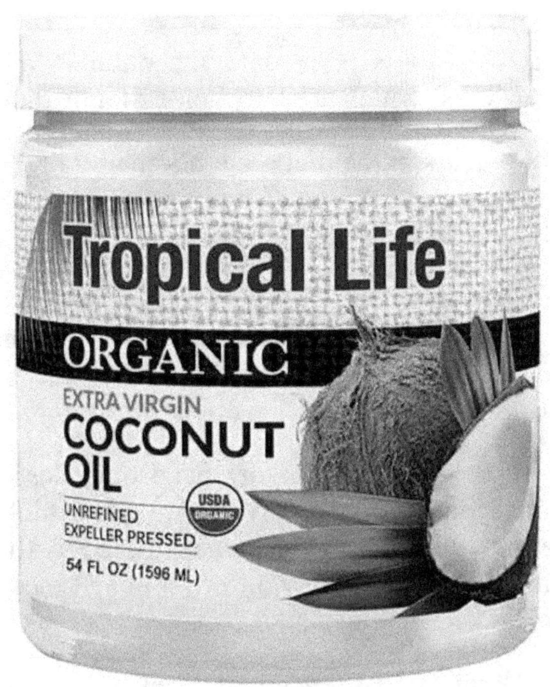

Tip #40
Put Coconut Oil in your body everyday

If there were one product on the market that I would recommend more than any other it would be Coconut Oil.

I am sold on it and highly recommend that *this outstanding source of great fat* be part of your daily diet, especially if you want to lose weight. There is not a day that goes by where I do not use this healthy product.

The benefits are way too long to list so to save time I would ask that you simply Google the impressive list of benefits that Coconut Oil has to offer.

Trust me when I say that this excellent source of fat (which we need) is in its own class. Coconut Oil contains Medium Chain Triglycerides (MCTs) which are fatty acids of a medium length.

Most of the fatty acids in the diet are long-chain fatty acids, but the medium-chain fatty acids in Coconut Oil are metabolized differently, which makes a world of difference.

The problem with most uniformed naysayers is that Coconut Oil will make you gain weight. Nothing could be further from the truth. In my opinion it is just the opposite, *and would highly recommend using this for anyone trying to lose weight.*

I personally use Coconut Oil for my Fat Bomb desserts (see Tip #33), as well as drench it on my real foods (think meats and vegetables) as an excellent sauce when mixed with real butter. Along with this I use it every day on my skin and face which takes away any dryness.

Your body and brain will rejoice and thank you when you begin feeding them with this outstanding source of fat. I also recommend it to any person who has Alzheimer's disease.

Remember that Coconut Oil contains a lot of medium chain triglycerides, which are metabolized differently and can have therapeutic effects on several brain disorders.

Here are ten quick and impressive benefits of Coconut Oil:

1. *Coconut Oil Contains Fatty Acids With Powerful Medicinal Properties.*

2. *Populations That Eat a Lot of Coconut Oil Are Healthy.*

3. *Coconut Oil Can Help You Burn More Fat.*

4. *Coconut Oil Can Kill Harmful Microorganisms.*

5. *Coconut Oil Can Reduce Your Hunger, Helping You Eat Less.*

6. *The Fatty Acids in Coconut Oil Are Turned into Ketones, Which Can Reduce Seizures.*

7. *Coconut Oil Can Improve Blood Cholesterol Levels.*

8. *Coconut Oil Can Protect Hair Against Damage, Moisturize Skin and Function as Sunscreen.*

9. *The Fatty Acids in Coconut Oil Can Boost Brain Function in Alzheimer's Patients.*

10. *Coconut Oil Can Help You Lose Fat, Especially The Harmful Abdominal Fat.*

My recommendation is to go with *Tropical Life Organic Extra Virgin Coconut Oil,* 54 fl oz. This can be purchased online (Walmart has had it online) and is much more affordable than purchasing it from a local grocery or health food store.

I love this brand not simply because of the outstanding price, but because it is extra virgin, unrefined, and expeller pressed. These are the qualities that you should look for in a Coconut Oil brand.

Bottom line: Start putting Coconut Oil in your body every day. You will LOVE the health benefits that it delivers!

"If there were one product on the market that I would recommend more than any other it would be Coconut Oil."

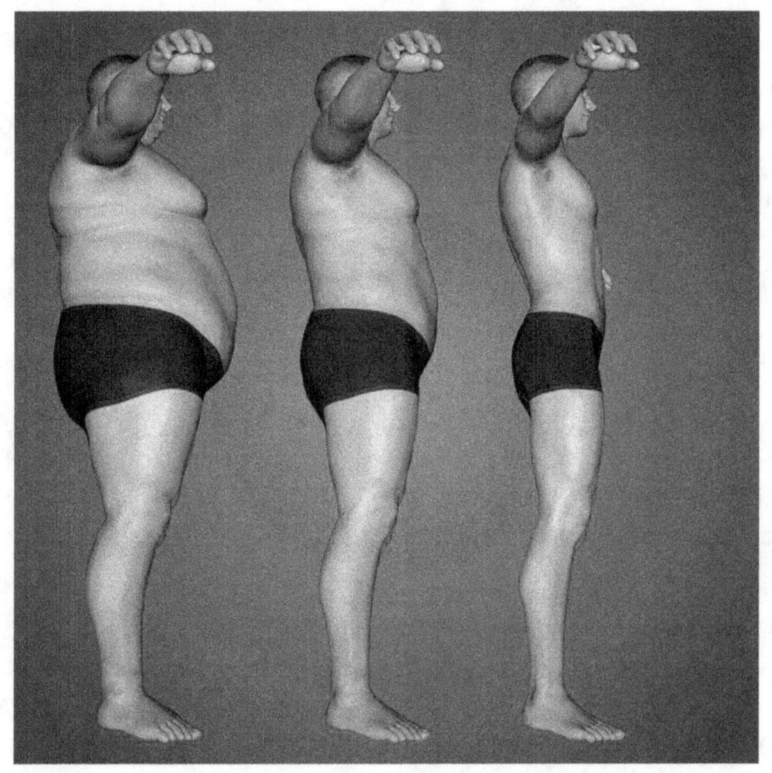

Tip #41
What I would do to lose 10, 20, 50, or 100+ pounds

Let me offer you the 3 things that I personally would do if I wanted to lose weight permanently.

The key word in the last sentence is PERMANENTLY as *I have no interest whatsoever in the hundreds of silly fad diets that eventually fail in the end.*

So here are my personal top three words of advice for losing weight permanently and would offer them to anyone who is tired of carrying around that extra weight:

#1 I WOULD LEARN TO EAT REAL FOOD

I have said this often throughout the book and will continue to give this advice: The majority of food (think boxed, bagged, canned or frozen) that is sitting on your friendly grocery store shelves is terrible for your waistline.

These are what I refer to as manufactured processed foods and are a major reason that you hate getting your picture taken. *These cheap products are here to stay since they are highly profitable for the big food manufacturers.*

Simply ask yourself prior to putting anything in your mouth *if 'ol Abe Lincoln would have eaten it.* In other words, our beloved 16th president more than likely ate REAL FOOD and that is the key to dropping weight permanently.

If you just began to avoid the vast majority of foods that are in a box, bag, can, or frozen, your weight would begin to drop simply because the vast majority of these foods are nothing more than refined carbs which quickly turn into sugar once they go into your body (think pastas), and then happily turn into fat cells on your body.

Here is a short list of food examples I am quite confident that 'ol Abe never ate:

- Corn dogs

- Lucky Charms (or any other boxed cereal)

- Pasta (any and all forms)

- Pop tarts

- Frozen dinners

- Fake cooking oils (terrible for the waistline)

- Sugary drinks (pops, juices, sugar laced teas)

- Pizza (sorry pizza lovers)

- Any type of chips in a bag

- And most everything else in a box, bag, can, or frozen.

If what you are about to put into your mouth could not have been found in 'ol Abe's kitchen, then more than likely it is fake food.

#2 I WOULD FLAT OUT QUIT MY ADDICTION TO SUGAR AND REFINED CARBS

This second tip alone will do wonders for any person's belly and hips as sugar and all of that processed food (which converts to sugar once it goes down the hatch) is the real culprit in keeping that extra weight on your body.

In order to lose weight you need to understand that all sugary foods (including our beloved sodas) *will make you fat eventually.*

By simply going cold turkey and eliminating sugar and refined carbs (think boxed pastas, potatoes, rice, corn, etc.), you will slowly begin to notice that your pants are getting baggier.

Listen, do not let anyone fool you into thinking you can have your cake and eat it too. *Sugar makes us fat, period.*

#3 I WOULD DO INTERMITTENT FASTING AS A LIFESTYLE

The final thing that I personally would do if I wanted to lose 10, 20, 50, or 100+ pounds would be to *live an Intermittent Fasting lifestyle* which is super easy and super healthy for your body.

Intermittent Fasting is simply not eating breakfast. That's it. It is giving your body up to 16-20 hours of fasting each day and allowing 6-8 hours for a feeding time window.

Most Intermittent Fasting follows this type of eating schedule:

Beginners:

- Eat between 12 pm and 8 pm

- This gives your body 16 hours of Intermittent Fasting

Advanced:

- Eat between 12 or 2 pm and 6 pm

- This gives your body 18-20 hours of Intermittent Fasting

Not only are the overall health benefits of Intermittent Fasting amazing, but the bonus benefit is that you will begin to notice your weight decreasing.

The key to Intermittent Fasting is to *stop believing Tony the Tiger and every breakfast food manufacturer out there* who has brainwashed our society into believing that breakfast is the most important meal of the day.

This may have been true 150 years ago when a majority of us were all farmers who worked 12-14 hours of manual labor, but it is simply not true today.

Trust me when I say that Intermittent Fasting works and your digestive system will thank you for the opportunity to rest from all the years of constantly shoving food into your body.

Your sad belly will definitely protest for the first week, but once you get past the loud growling and moaning you will soon realize that Intermittent Fasting is really quite easy, especially now that you are staying fuller for longer *due to eating real foods*.

So in review, I personally would do the following 3 things if I wanted to lose weight and keep it off permanently:

#1 I would learn to eat REAL FOOD and divorce all processed foods.

#2 I would divorce sugar COMPLETELY from my life (Sorry Little Debbies which by the way use to be my favorite!).

#3 I would make Intermittent Fasting a permanent lifestyle.

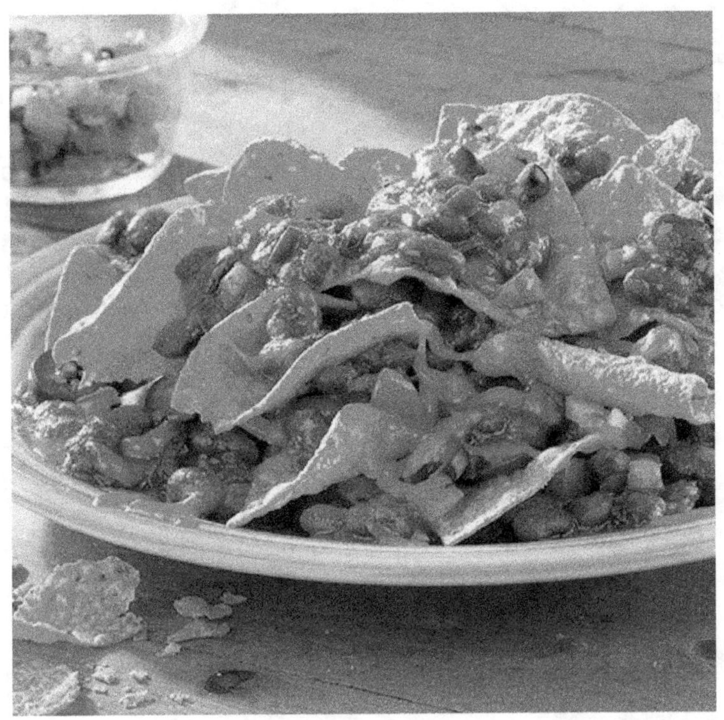

Tip #42
Stop buying appetizers if you want to lose weight

I remember in the past when this new concept called "Appetizers" began finding its way into the menus of restaurants throughout our great land.

It was capitalism at its finest and a great business move for the deep pockets of restaurant owners, and continues to make major bucks for every restaurant out there.

This new appetizer experiment was soon here to stay and eventually brainwashed the masses of innocent restaurant patrons into believing that *a meal was not complete unless they first stuffed their faces with a greasy fat producing appetizer.*

But seriously, I really do not get it and in my life cannot count on my left hand how many times I have actually ordered one of these fried, heart attack promoting trans fat appetizers.

The majority of appetizers is absolutely terrible for you and is dripping with the fats that you definitely do not want in your body.

But you have to love the names that they put on these fat belly producing foods. Listen to some of Chili's cool names that they list on their appetizer menu:

- Honey-Chipotle Crispers® & Waffles (will make you fat)

- Loaded Boneless Wings (again, will make you fat)

- Southwestern Eggrolls (will make you fat)

- California Grilled Chicken Flatbread (will make you fat)

- Classic Nachos with Fajita Chicken (will make you fat)

- Chips & Salsa (ask the waitress what the chips are fried in)

- Fried Pickles (will make you fat)

All and every one of the above appetizers will make you fat *(did I already mention that?)* and should be avoided at all costs.

And by the way, the only appetizer that I would get from Chili's (or any other restaurant for that manner) is simply a bowl of Guacamole, and that is it.

No offense to any of you appetizer lovers out there, but my advice is to use the ten bucks that you would be wasting and go spend it on a deluxe super duper wash with wax at your local car wash instead.

The bottom line is this: *All appetizers are bad for your hips and belly and will eventually make any person overweight.* If it were my choice I would change the name on all of the menus out there from Appetizers to Fatetizers.

If you really want to become healthier then get all restaurant appetizers completely out of your life. Your trimmer body and shiny washed car will appreciate it.

"*If you really want to become healthier then get all restaurant appetizers completely out of your life.*"

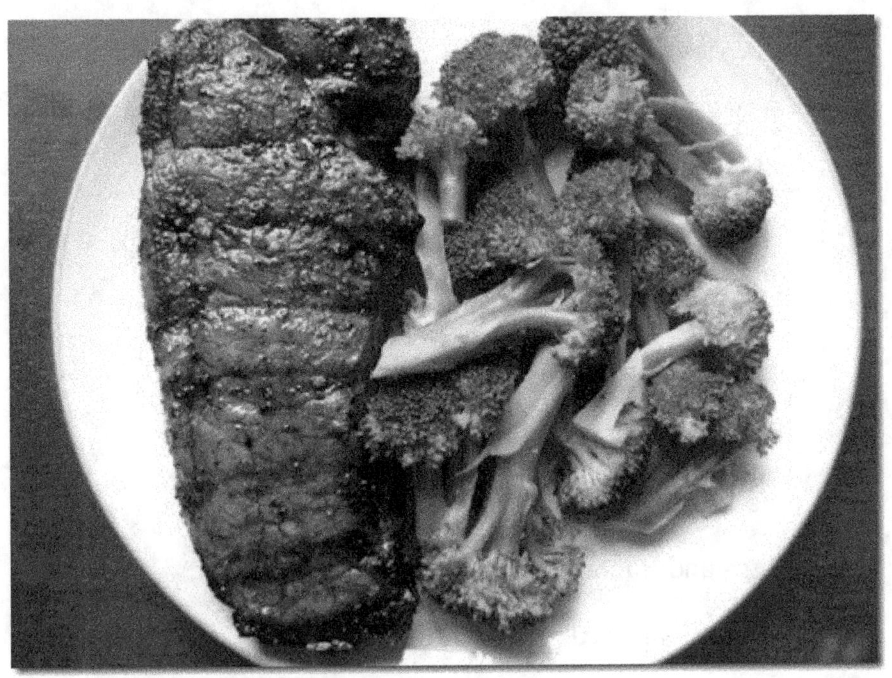

Tip #43
What I would order on a typical restaurant menu

So you are excited about doing a complete makeover from living decades munching on the myriads of fake foods that flood our land and have decided to venture into a new healthier lifestyle by eating REAL FOODS.

Sure it is easy to control what goes into your mouth in the comforts of your own kitchen, *but how do you handle it when you are going to a restaurant with family and friends?*

Let me show you what I would recommend and not recommend on any typical restaurant menu in order to stay healthy and lean:

RECOMMENDED:

- Any vegetable drenched in REAL butter *(yes REAL butter)*

- Most meats

- Hamburger (without the bun or sugar laced ketchup)

- Most Salads (avoid fat producing croutons)

- Chicken (not fried)

- Fajitas (for Mexican food lovers - careful on the tortillas)

- Fish (not fried)

- Eggs and Bacon

- Water, Plain Tea, or Black Coffee

AVOID LIKE THE BLACK PLAGUE:

- ALL fried foods (sorry French fry lovers)

- Most Sauces Including BBQ Sauce (it is just glorified sugar)

- ALL Breads (unless you want instant weight gain)

- Pancakes (which are really only sponges for the sugary syrup)

- Potatoes, Rice, Corn (all turns to sugar in your body)

- ALL Pastas (your body only recognizes it as sugar)

- Noodles (converts to sugar)

- ALL Sugar Drinks (it is simply water, sugar, and sticky syrup)

- Desserts (only on special occasions)

Becoming healthy again is really quite simple and comes down to the food choices that you are making.

So become aware that in most restaurants *you do have the option to make a wise food choice* that will not throw off your new healthy eating lifestyle.

"*Becoming healthy again is really quite simple and comes down to the food choices that you are making.*"

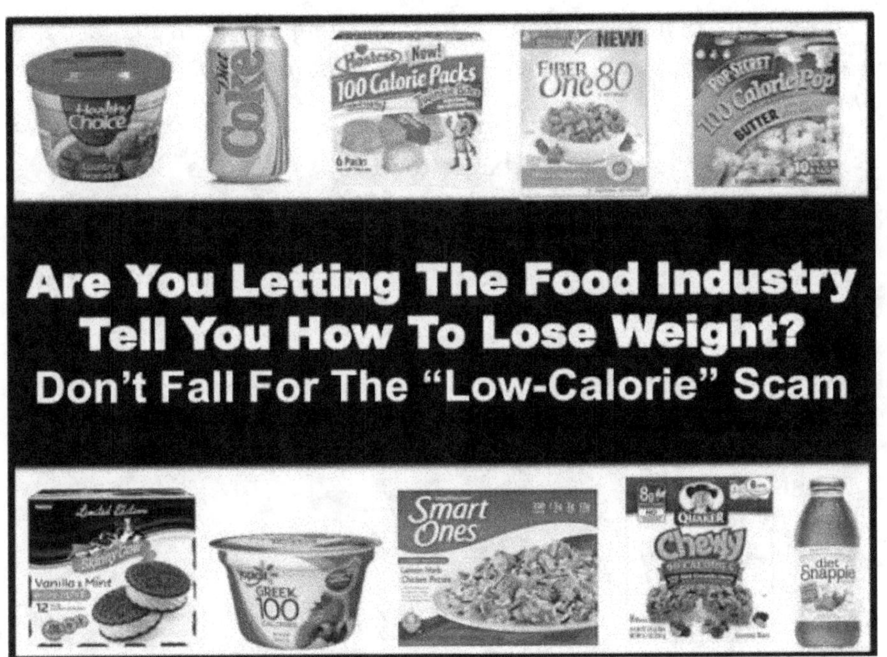

Tip #44
Recognize the low calorie food scam

Don't be deceived by the hundreds of food items on the grocery shelves proudly telling you that they are healthy, low in calories, and that you will get leaner by putting them into your belly.

It is all a complete scam and these types of manufactured foods are terrible for you. Stop making your "trying to lose weight" decisions be based on the silly concept known as calorie counting.

You will not lose weight when your whole diet strategy is based on the brainwashed concept known as the popular calorie in vs. calorie out crazy belief. *What matters the most in losing weight is the quality of the food you are eating, period.*

This eating low calorie garbage food is a completely wrong strategy and is seriously unhealthy for any person because you are basing your selection of food *not on whether the food choices are healthy for you, but by the silly amount of calories that it is proudly displaying.*

I mean really, a total garbage food like Hostess Twinkies is bragging on their box that it only has 100 calories in each pack? So like innocent sheep heading to the slaughter, dieters grab a couple of boxes of Twinkies because it fits into their silly daily calorie counting diet program.

And how can a garbage product like Yoplait Greek Yogurt not be ashamed of itself by proudly announcing to the world that it only contains 100 calories, when in reality it is simply a sugar laced fattening dessert?

Listen real carefully to what I am about to say:

If you really want to become leaner then remember that more important than anything else is whether the food is REAL FOOD.

In other words, it all depends on the QUALITY of what you are eating and not on the silly calories that these fake foods loudly boast about on their colorful labels.

Do not fall for the calorie game as the real key in getting that weight off can only happen *when you stop eating all of these terrible fake foods* and simply learn to eat real food.

On a personal note, I have never counted calories as it is a complete waste of time in my opinion. What is not a waste of time is learning to simply eat real food and watch as your weight begins to drop.

The majority of foods that come from a box, bag, can, or frozen is made in a factory and is the culprit that will eventually make you gain weight.

Stop being deceived by these low calorie grocery store items as they are detrimental to your health. *Choose instead what your body craves, and that is REAL FOOD.*

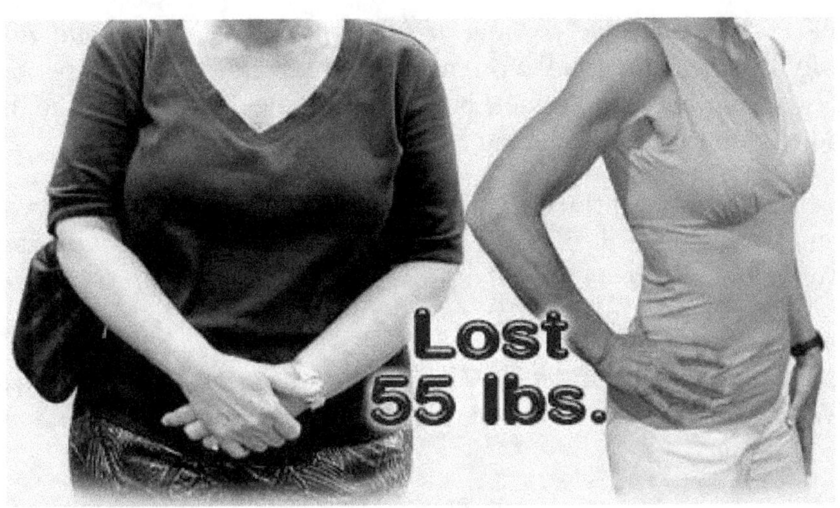

Tip #45
Choose either sugar or a healthier body

Whenever a person approaches and asks what I believe is "the secret" to becoming healthier my first and foremost response is always the same:

I simply say to quit sugar.

The immediate response to this simple answer is usually the same for most people and that is that *they proudly proclaim that they love sugar to much*, or they can never imagine life without candy and sweets.

So I just smile and show grace as I listen to this typical response from those who may genuinely want to become healthier or sincerely want to lose weight.

So let me share what I believe is the real issue with the majority of those who are desperately seeking an answer *to permanent weight loss.*

You cannot continue to have a love affair with sugar and lose weight at the same time. You must choose one or the other, period. It is a plain and simple fact, but hard on the ears of those who are addicted to this fat producing toxin.

Let me be straightforward on this touchy subject. Unless you completely get rid of consistently eating sugar you will stay overweight. *Sugar is the #1 reason that the majority of Americans are either overweight or obese.*

For many within our society, sugar is at the center of their lives. Every happy event or celebration revolves around our beloved toxic friend.

Whether it is Billy's 10th birthday party or the office party celebration, our sweet little friend sugar is the main guest waiting to be gobbled up.

So it is your choice and your choice alone on the matter of sugar. *Stay with it and continue to hold weight, or run as fast as you can from this deadly toxin and watch your weight begin to disappear.*

get fit in the gym lose weight IN THE KITCHEN

Tip #46
Weight loss occurs in the kitchen, not the gym

Here is the typical game plan for many hopefuls who finally get tired of carrying around that extra weight and decide that the gym is the answer to shedding the poundage:

Couple A and B go and purchase a new pair of sneakers, buy cute matching outfits (with the swoosh on it), join a local gym, and begin their weight loss journey that will hopefully one day lead them to the promise land of Leanville.

Soon after the Christmas tree is taken down there are usually a large number of enthusiasts who will begin migrating to the gym after gorging on an embarrassing amount of cookies during the holiday season. Their game plan is to look like those lean models on television trying to sell you that $2,499.00 ski machine thing.

I really do commend anyone who is motivated to fork over the money for the new gym membership, *but the sad truth is that a high percentage will eventually drift away by the time February 1st rolls around.*

I once heard a person say that a six pack can only be made in the kitchen. Let me add to that... *Weight loss can only happen in the kitchen as well.*

Sure you can lose a pound or two here and there huffing and puffing as you do your thing in the gym, but if you are not completely changing your bad food diet to a good food diet *(or REAL FOOD)*, then you are basically wasting your time in a vain attempt to shed the weight.

Yes, I do understand that exercise has some really great benefits, but losing weight is not one of them...that is only reserved for the kitchen.

A very small percentage of your weight loss will occur in the gym and that is about it. A super large (90% +) of whether or not you succeed will be determined by what is at the end of your spoon and fork. *No ifs, ands, or buts about it.* It is the kitchen that you really need to focus on if you want to lose the weight.

Go to any gym on the planet and you will see a large segment of the population sweating up a storm on the various machines *in a desperate attempt to shed the pounds.* That is great and again I commend them for this.

But as for myself I often wonder if all of these people are as diligent with their selection of food choices as they are in the gym huffing away.

Again, I would highly encourage any person to exercise as it is great for your overall health. But please understand that any serious weight loss *is primarily found in the kitchen.*

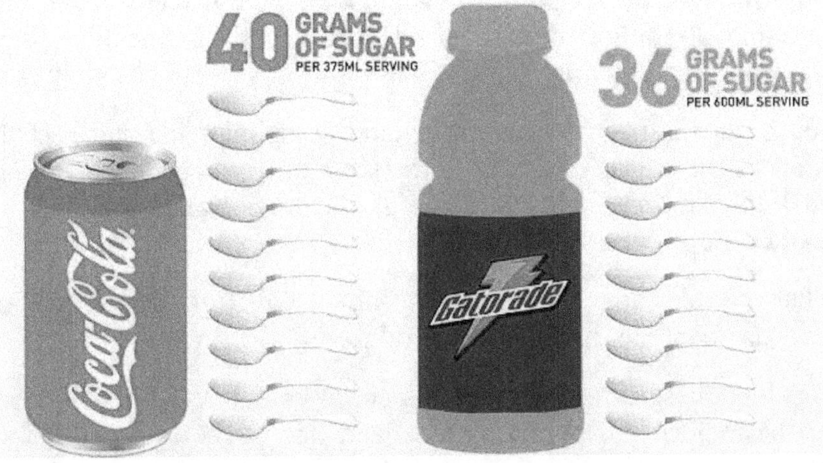

Tip #47
Sports drinks and "health" bars are bad for you

It is amazing how slick advertisement has totally brainwashed our society into believing that sports drinks like Gatorade and the dozens of so-called health bars lining the shelves somehow are excellent for our health.

Here is my advice...

Stay as far away from them as they are NOT HEALTHY choices at all.

Yes, I am aware of those Gatorade commercials featuring the billion dollar superstar athletes gulping down a bottle of blue liquid and then trying to convince us that they are great at their sport due in large part to this glorified colored sugar drink.

We also tend to forget the major bucks that these athletes are raking in for an easy day's work by simply smiling into the camera and drinking the blue stuff. I mean just imagine if you were offered a couple of million dollars just to smile and sip the blue sugar water...*pretty tempting isn't it?*

I have zero issue with capitalism and companies making a profit. But let's be real on this subject. *These sports drinks are nothing more than sugar, water, salt, and a few other ingredients that are hard to pronounce.*

What people are really purchasing is *all the hype* that the advertisement has successfully produced.

Guzzling these types of drinks is simply sideline Kool-Aid treats for the majority of young athletes and one of the reasons that we have obesity in our youth. If their favorite pro sport star can drink the blue stuff, *then it must be good enough for little Billy and his fifth grade buddies as well!*

Gatorade's 32 ounce Thirst Quencher contains a whopping 56 grams of sugar (14 teaspoons!) and a regular Gatorade has 36 grams of sugar (9 teaspoons!).

Trust me when I say that all of these types of sports drinks will eventually make you fat as well as mess up your body with all of that sugar storing away in your fat cells.

The same can be said about the majority of the so-called health bars with the appearance of being a healthy alternative.

Most are terrible for your body and convert to sugar once they enter your system. Also, see how many words you can pronounce on the small ingredient list on the back of many of these product packages.

If you are serious about getting your health back then I would personally advice you to totally separate yourself from any and all sugar laced "sports" drinks as well as the majority of the so-called health bars that in my opinion are simply glorified candy bars.

Your body will thank you for it.

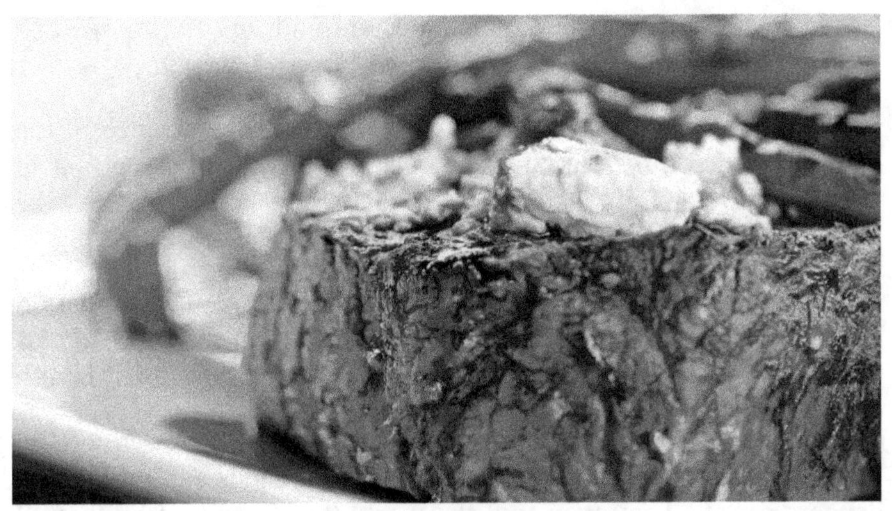

Tip #48
Give me the fat on my hamburger and steak

An amazing declaration happened in the 1960's that not only has contributed to us becoming an obese nation, but this declaration also had opened the door to accepting the dangerous cooking oils that are in most kitchen cabinets today (names like Crisco, Mazola, Wesson, and Smart balance).

And what was the announcement that assisted in making us fat as well as accept unhealthy cooking oils with open arms? It was loudly declared to the world that all fats were now an enemy to your health and would cause all kinds of terrible diseases.

The sad truth even today is that *the majority of people still believes this warped science* from decades ago and still holds fast that fats (especially animal fats) will make you sick and fat.

I use to be in that camp where I would buy the leanest steaks and make sure all of the fat was cut off prior to throwing it on the grill. You would never catch me eating any animal fat or chicken skin.

Now I laugh at my past silly uneducated mind *and so happy to be set free to now enjoy the juiciest, fat laced steaks around.*

Let me get to the point. If you are still stuck in the science of the 1960's my recommendation is to reeducate yourself by going to Google and learn about how our bodies need fats in order to be healthy.

Think about it. For thousands of years mankind from every nation has eaten animal fat without having an ounce of guilt. Then all of a sudden a few men in white laboratory coats and bad breath declared to the world that all fats were evil.

So what happened after this breaking news decades ago on the evil dangers of fat? They then told the world that fats like lard that all of your ancestors cooked with for centuries were dangerous and instead you needed to start using these unhealthy cooking oils like Crisco and Wesson Oil.

This in my opinion has become one of the worst health moves that mankind has ever made.

You would be hard pressed to find real convincing evidence that truly shows that animal fat is either bad for you or will make you fat. The real enemy to your health is trans fats and all of those fake cooking oils in clear bottles that line the shelves at your friendly grocery store. *This is the real enemy to your health and heart.*

And please do not believe the little heart sign that is displayed on their clear bottled labels. Consuming any of these manufactured cooking oils will eventually make you very unhealthy.

I personally love animal fat and no, it does not make us fat. On the flip side, eating lean meats do not make us "lean".

We have a twisted mindset by somehow equating that eating fats will make us fat and eating lean meats will make us lean. Nothing could be further from the truth.

As an interesting side note, when a pack of lions go in for the kill they look for the fat on the dead animal first and have very little interest in the lean meat. *I somewhat believe that these lions understand the importance of fats better than we do.*

Give me the fattest hamburger meat, the juiciest marbled fat steak, and the fattest cut of bacon out of the bunch. I will take five skin covered chicken legs fried in bacon grease over a dry and terrible tasting white chicken breast any day of the year.

If bacon grease was good enough for 'ol Abe Lincoln, then it is good enough for me. *Why the majority of people use these fake and dangerous manufactured cooking oils in a bottle is beyond me.*

I personally now crave animal fat as it totally fills me up and keeps me full *for a very long time.* It is the fat that makes all of these meats so tasty, and no it does not cause heart disease or clog your arteries.

The evidence is simply not there. The real culprit is these fake cooking oils and trans fats that are dangerous to our health. Simply learn more about this topic by going to Google and researching it.

You just need to stop drinking the Kool-Aid presented by those laboratory guys with the thick glasses from the 60's and enter the 21st century of science. Again, go to Google and learn why it is perfectly safe and healthy to eat fats.

Since eating fats I think more clearly *and never have a craving for junk food.* And trust me when I say that not one ounce of any of this animal fat has put an ounce of fat on me.

I look back at all those wasted years of depriving myself of all of those delicious cuts of fat meat that I banned from my mouth. *How foolish was I to think I was eating healthy with my dry and tasteless white chicken breast.*

If you cannot get over the government's decades of brainwashing and war against eating fats *I totally get it* as I was once a citizen in your camp of dried steak and chicken.

But those days are gone simply because I stepped out of the science from the 1960's, stopped drinking the Kool-Aid, and entered the 21st century.

Since bringing fats back into my life I cannot tell you how much more healthy my body feels and how focused I am when performing a task.

Now everyday feels like a beautiful banquet for me with the complete freedom from any guilt to enjoy fat and juicy hamburgers (without the bun), marble laced steaks, and thick cut fat bacon.

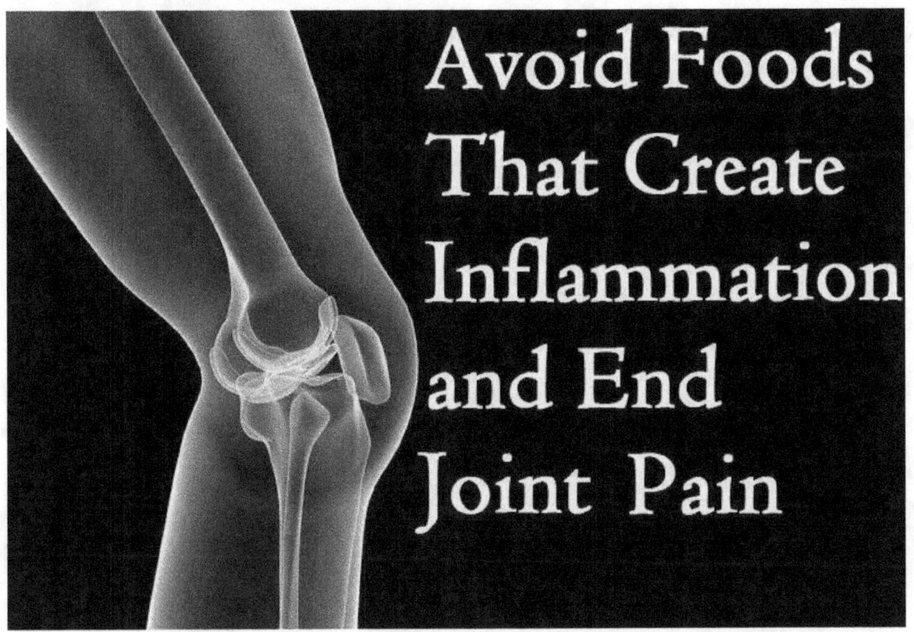

Tip #49
Sugar may be the real cause of joint pain

I often wonder deep inside whenever I hear a person complaining about the trials of growing older with joint pains and inflammatory issues, and then declaring to anyone who will listen that it is "just a part of aging".

For some reason I just have a hard time wrapping my head around the common belief that with aging automatically comes the moans and groans of painful joints or arthritis.

Let me give you my personal take on this issue that more than likely you *will never hear* from your friendly doctor who instead offers you prescription drugs that really is just an expensive bandage to the real issue.

I personally believe joint pain and arthritis is simply a result of years of abusing your body with sugar and refined carbs (fake foods).

Understand this important point: *Our bodies were never meant to be stuffed with this toxin known as sugar along with the myriads of fake food in a box that populate our friendly grocery store shelves.*

My view for a majority of these inflammatory pain issues is that *it is the poor selection of foods* that you have abused your body with for decades that is the real culprit to this problem.

I would compare it to always putting bad gas into your car and then one day wondering why the car won't start.

So let me give anyone who is continually fighting an inflammatory pain issue some advice: *Stop eating sugar and the majority of foods that are found in a box, bag, can, or frozen.*

Have some patience since you more than likely have abused your body for decades following the Standard American Diet (or SAD Diet). Allow all of that garbage *to slowly get out of your system* and then see if your inflammatory problems begin to dissipate.

And trust me when I say that more than likely your friendly doctor with his framed degrees proudly hanging in his office will not give you this advice. *Why in the world would he want to lose a patient?*

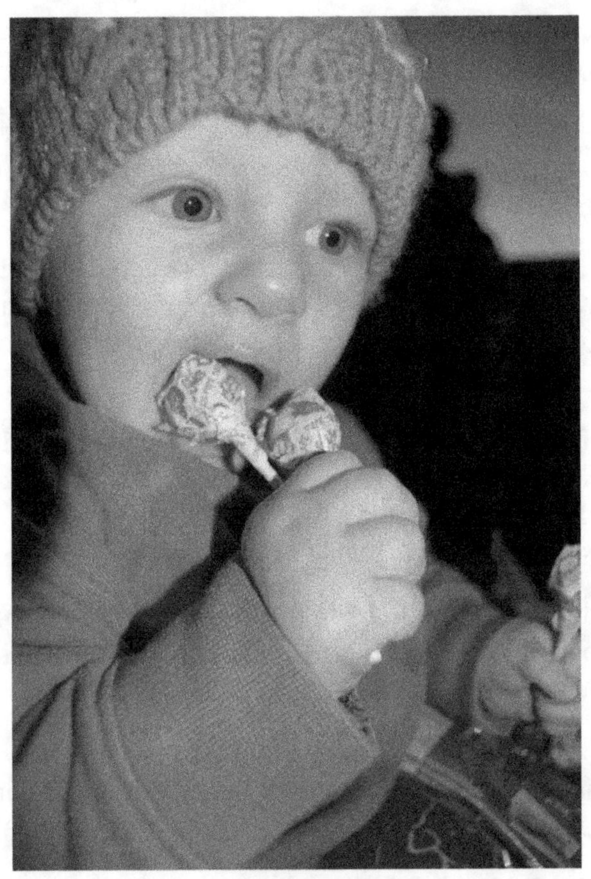

Tip #50
Beloved Sugar: The sacred cow most will not leave

I have come to learn that of all the food items that our bellies take pleasure in, no food even comes close to our beloved sugar.

Talk to almost anyone on the serious and damaging effects of consuming sugar and you are sure to get crossed arms and a defiant look.

It has been said that the two topics that should never be discussed are politics and religion (which I disagree).

But I have come to understand that there is also a third topic that should never be discussed, *and that is the dangers of consuming sugar.*

Here is my view on why very few would (or could) ever leave this sacred cow. From our earliest memories most of us have viewed sugar as our secret best friend and major source of comfort (outside of our little stuffed teddy bear).

As an adorable two year cute child you fell and scraped your little knee. So what does mommy do? She plugs your little mouth with a little Dum Dums sucker and all of a sudden your pain disappears *with the rush of pure sugar entering your system.*

From that day forward you soon discover that all sorts of problems could temporarily be forgotten by simply putting this perfectly legal substance into your body.

Feeling depressed? Grab a frosted cupcake or eat a bowl of Lucky Charms *(use to be my favorite)* and the depression instantly leaves for a few minutes.

Feeling lonely? You have discovered that nothing comforts and temporarily takes the loneliness away better than a box of Little Debbies *(my favorite use to be yummy Swiss Miss Cake Rolls).*

So I do get it. I also recognize that the majority within our society would never even consider leaving their trusted pal, *especially after all the happy memories that this toxin has brought into their lives.*

Statistics state that the average person in America consumes around 150 pounds of sugar a year. That is about 3 pounds every week which personally is staggering to grasp.

In closing, I have been there and was also a part of the *Sugar Lovers Club* for many years and would never truly admit that I was addicted to the stuff.

But as a closing testimonial since divorcing this longtime pal, I have never felt better or had my brain be able to think more clearly as it does today.

For years I had heard the various stories of the brave few who had permanently left sugar for good and not only lost tons of weight, but felt so much healthier.

I only wish that I would have listened to their advice earlier.

"Talk to almost anyone on the serious and damaging effects of consuming sugar and you are sure to get crossed arms and a defiant look."

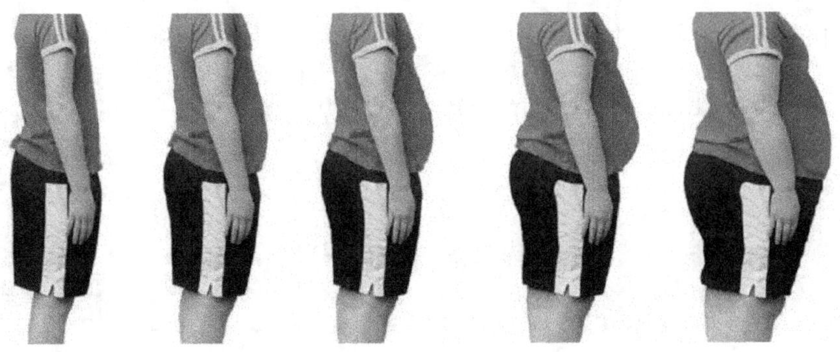

Tip #51
Why your belly and hips keep getting bigger

Let me get straight to the point on something that probably has been bothering you for years. You continue to try all of the silly diets out there and still the results are that you hate looking in a mirror and getting your picture taken.

Here is your real problem, and nothing more:

For the vast majority it is because you have a terrible diet and more than likely are clueless to this fact. The deceptive label on the box of food you just ate last night advertises that it is a "healthy choice", but in reality is a fake food that will keep weight on.

More than likely the food choices that you have made in the past and continue to make are the real reason that your clothes continue to get smaller. If what you are eating is not REAL FOOD *but instead made in a manufacturing plant,* then it will be difficult to maintain a healthy weight.

Not to burst anybody's bubble, but our bodies were never designed to carry all of that extra weight that the majority of Americans are slowly tugging around. *Being obese is abnormal and poor food choices are the #1 reason that you may be fighting this issue.*

My personal interest in writing on this topic is that I recognize that being overweight puts a major cramp in a person's quality of life. The simple things that a healthy person takes for granted like walking in a park is lost for someone who cannot due to a weight issue.

As an example, a few months ago I was in a Walmart and coming down my narrow aisle was a very obese young woman in a riding scooter. My heart immediately went out to her as I tried to imagine how daily life must have been for her. *It is in moments like these that tug at my heart.*

Again, it is all about the poor choices of foods that you may have been eating for decades that more than likely have brought you to where you are at today.

My word of encouragement is please do not give up as this can be reversible by simply reeducating yourself in what REAL FOOD is *(what 'ol Abe Lincoln would have ate),* divorcing sugar, and eliminating the majority of foods found in a box, bag, can, or frozen.

Stop going on silly diets and decide today to make a complete lifestyle change in the way that you eat *(think REAL FOOD)* and the weight will eventually begin to disappear for good.

It is your decision alone and the only thing that you will have to look forward to in the near future is seeing a new and healthy person staring back at you in the mirror.

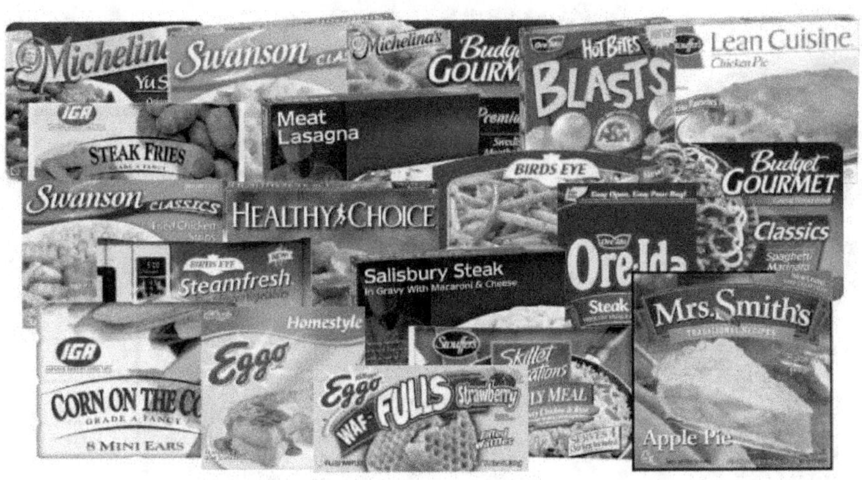

Tip #52
10 foods to banish from your diet

#1

Avoid all cereals

#2

Avoid all manufactured cooking oils

#3

Avoid all fruit juices (including 100% juice)

#4

Avoid breads, bagels, & crackers

#5

Avoid most foods that are boxed, bagged, canned, or frozen

#6

Avoid all forms of pasta

#7

Avoid all types of sugar (including honey)

#8

Avoid most condiments such as ketchup and BBQ

#9

Avoid fried foods

#10

Avoid cookies, candies, desserts

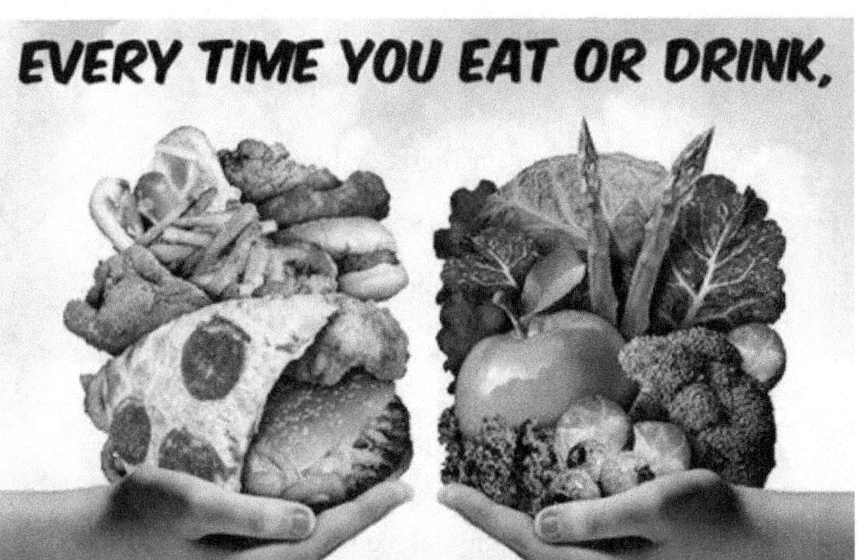

Tip #53
My 10 favorite health tips

#10

Stop sitting all the time and start an exercise program

#9

Simply ask yourself if 'ol Abe Lincoln would have eaten it

#8

Eat foods that keep your insulin low

#7

Make wise choices when visiting a restaurant

#6

Make Intermittent Fasting a daily part of your life

#5

Stop drinking all fruit juices

#4

Put coconut oil in your body everyday (think Fat Bombs)

#3

Stay away from anything labeled "low fat" or "no fat"

#2

Eat healthy fats everyday

#1

Stay away from all sugars and processed foods

Additional Resources

Here are a few additional online resources for improving your health:

www.dietdoctor.com

This is an outstanding website with 100's of great resources on the low carb lifestyle.

Butter Bob Briggs

www.buttermakesyourpantsfalloff.com

Butter Bob was the person who opened my eyes to the importance of putting fats back into our diets and the importance of keeping our insulin low.

Bob has some outstanding videos online. My recommendation would to go to www.youtube.com and watch these five videos to learn more:

Butter Bob Must Watch YouTube Video Titles:

Butter Makes Your Pants Fall Off (29:02)

The Root of Modern Illness – High Insulin (25:56)

At the Store with Butter Bob (14:22)

You Got to Get Sugar Out of Your Life (13:56)

You are Either Fed or Fasted (9:29)

Here is a before and after picture of Butter Bob

(Went from 320 pounds to 175 pounds in 14 months!)

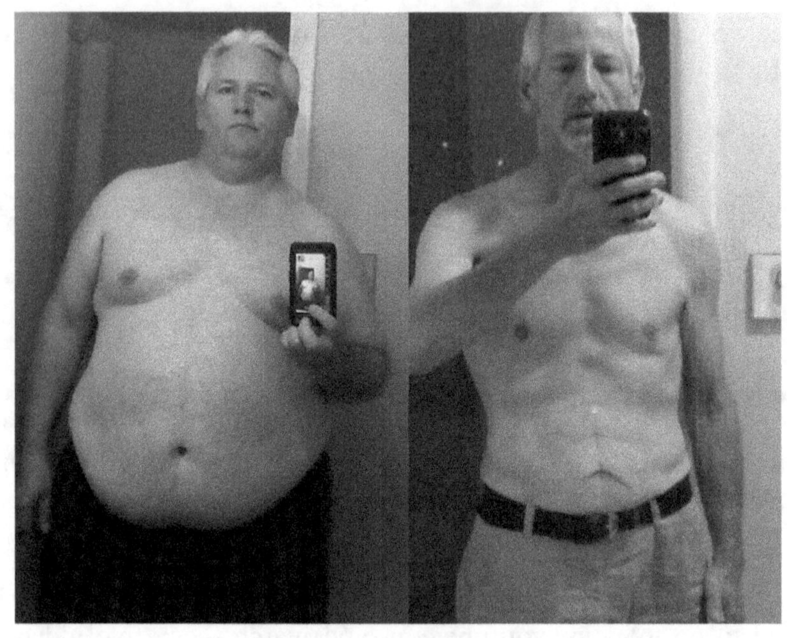

Check out a few other great YouTube video presenters:

Dr. Robert H. Lustig

Sugar: The Bitter Truth (129:00)

Dr. Eric Berg

Dr. Eric Westman

Dr. Jason Fung

Dr. Andreas Eenfeldt

Dr. Tim Noakes

Gary Taubes

Go Keto with Casey

Book a Speaking Seminar

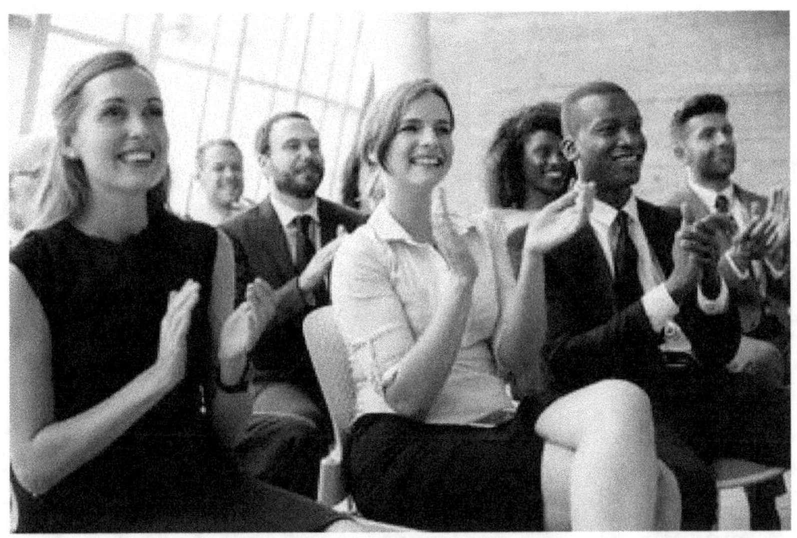

Looking for a fun and educational health seminar for your next event?

If you would like to book Cary at your next meeting on the topic of improving your overall health, then please visit us at:

www.roadtobetterhealth.net

Whether your next event revolves around offering a health seminar for your workplace, upcoming expo or conference, church or civic club, or any other type of social group, our *Road to Better Health Seminars* are a perfect fit to educate your audience *on how to feel better, lose weight, and think clearer.* Contact us today at **www.roadtobetterhealth.net**.